The EMDR Coloring Book II

The EMDR Coloring Book II
A Calming Resource for Adults
Featuring 100 Works of Art
Paired With
100 Positive Affirmations

Mark Odland - MA, LMFT, MDIV

Bilateral Innovations
Minnesota

Published in the United States by Bilateral Innovations
www.bilateralinnovations.com
mark@bilateralinnovations.com

Artwork printed with permission from the National Gallery of Art.

Names: Odland, Mark, author.
Title: The EMDR Coloring Book: A Calming Resource for Adults Featuring 100 Works of Art Paired with 100 Positive Affirmations
Description: First American edition. Minnesota: Bilateral Innovations, an assumed name of North Woods Christian Counseling, LLC, [2018]
BISAC: Medical / Mental Health

ISBN-13:   9781985209176
ISBN-10:   1985209179

Content available as a Paperback Book.

PRINTED IN THE UNITED STATES OF AMERICA

10 9 8 7 6 5 4 3 2 1

First American Edition

PREFACE

Who this Book is for

While this book could be enjoyed by almost anyone, it's designed specifically for those receiving EMDR therapy. If you're in this process, your therapist may have already helped you develop resources like a "safe place," "calm place," or "container." Often used before or after EMDR therapy, these resources can also be a wonderful way to practice emotional regulation between sessions. The EMDR Coloring Book is designed to complement these strategies, providing you with another resource for the journey.

Whether you choose to use crayons, markers, colored pencils, or paint, this "coloring book" will help you practice being in the moment. A break from past hurts and future worries, this book provides an opportunity to reclaim the curious and playful parts of yourself. Paired with positive self-statements, each work of art invites thoughtful meditation on the truths so many of us hope to believe as the healing process unfolds.

When to Use this Book

This book could be useful in situations where you would like to:

1) Center yourself before, during, or at the end of an EMDR therapy session.
2) Practice emotional regulation between EMDR therapy sessions.
3) Relax at home or on the road.
4) Enjoy beautiful and thought-provoking artwork.
5) Meditate on positive self-statements.
6) Rediscover the the playful and curious side of yourself.

How to Use this Book

Choose your medium to create with

You may use crayons, colored pencils, markers, watercolor paints, or any other creative medium that feels right for you. Some find it helpful to journal or jot down ideas next to the images. Others will create a collage. There are no rules with this book, so feel free to "color outside the lines."

Stage your environment

When used at home, you might consider eliminating distractions and arranging your environment to be visually beautiful and emotionally peaceful (light candles, play soothing music, etc.). When used outside the home, this may not be possible. However, when on the move, this book's portability allows it to be used in a therapist's office, at a park, on a bus, or anywhere you see fit.

Use as part of a larger self-care plan

While this book is helpful to use as needed for practicing mindfulness and relaxation, you might also consider using it as part of a larger self-care plan. With busy schedules, taking care of ourselves can be challenging. However, taking even small steps to add beauty, love, and peace into our lives can make a big difference over time. By investing just a few minutes a day, coloring and journaling could become an enjoyable addition to your daily or weekly routine.

Select a page to interact with and begin

As you begin to color or paint, consider being mindful of how the image and positive statement associated with it impacts you. If thinking about the positive statement leads to pleasant emotions, simply notice these feelings and continue. If this focus leads to unsettling emotions that are tolerable, you can either choose to color, paint, or journal your way "through them," or instead redirect your focus back to your surroundings and to the creative process... simply noticing the weight of the object in your hand, the texture of the paper, and the various colors as they emerge. Let yourself go with the flow, allowing yourself to simply respond rather than overthinking it. Of course, you are free to finish at any time.

Disclaimer

* This book is designed to be relaxing. It may provide you with a much needed break from the stress of life, and an opportunity to be more fully-present in the moment. For most, the tactile nature of the creative process tends to be grounding. However, if for some reason the process becomes upsetting or leads to emotions that are too difficult to manage, you can always stop. Simply stand-up, take deep breaths, move your body, engage your senses, and utilize your coping skills. While the book can be used as a resource during the EMDR therapy process, it is not to be confused with EMDR therapy itself, which should only be provided by a trained EMDR therapist. When using this book, make sure to talk with your therapist to confirm it aligns with your treatment goals.

How the Positive Affirmations were Selected

The positive self-statements in this book were inspired by the positive "cognitions" listed in EMDR therapy basic trainings. These core affirmations and their variants are familiar to EMDR therapists around the world because they depict the types of statements clients want to believe as they heal from their trauma. While some of these statements might not technically meet the definition of a "cognition," they've been included because of their potential to be helpful and encouraging.

How the Artwork was Chosen

In contrast to the first EMDR Coloring Book, for this new book I intentionally selected images that would be less thought-provoking, and even more emotionally neutral. I therefore eliminated images depicting people and introduced mandalas, Celtic knots, floral designs, and other geometric artwork from publicdomainvectors.com. My hope is that the simple designs will allow you to "get lost" in the coloring process and enjoy the art of "just noticing." Another notable change is that unlike the first book, now images are only printed on one side, allowing you to cut or rip out individual pages. I sincerely hope that you enjoy using this book, and that it plays some small role in your process of healing.

Blessings,

Mark Odland - MA, LMFT, MDIV

CONTENTS

99	I can trust my judgment
101	I am safe now
103	I deserve love
105	I can be present
107	I can learn to trust myself
109	I deserve to live
111	I am not alone
113	I am able to succeed
115	I am worthy of love
117	I can be trusted
119	I am honorable
121	I have dignity
123	I am valuable
125	I am stronger than before
127	I am fine as I am
129	I am only human
131	I am smart
133	I am whole
135	I can handle it
137	I am enough
139	I can be myself
141	I can make mistakes
143	I am intelligent
145	I am strong now
147	I can be healthy
149	I am a work in progress
151	I do the best I can
153	I have been made new
155	I am okay just the way I am
157	I am strong
159	I can do it
161	I am forgiven
163	I have what it takes
165	I am okay as I am
167	I am a soulful person
169	I can accomplish my goals
171	I am valuable the way I am
173	I am not defined by my past
175	I have mastery
177	I did enough
179	I can be free
181	I can make good decisions
183	I am alright
185	I am lovely
187	I am remarkable

I am…

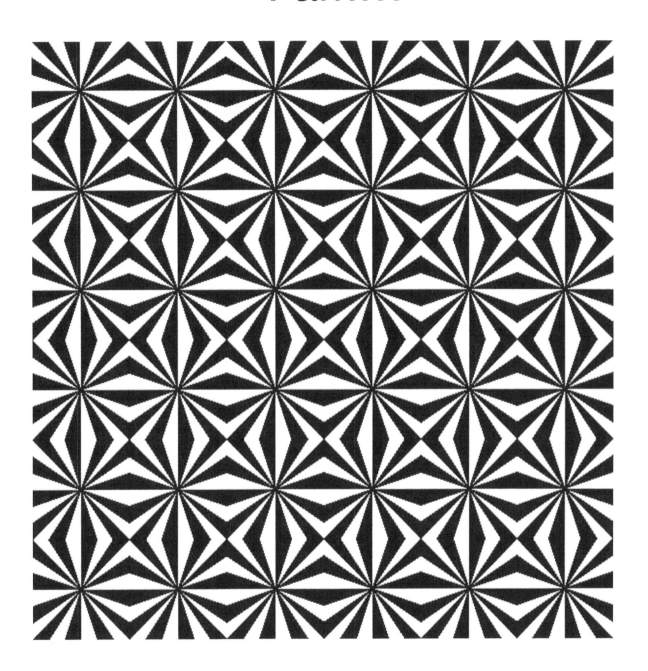

I am loved

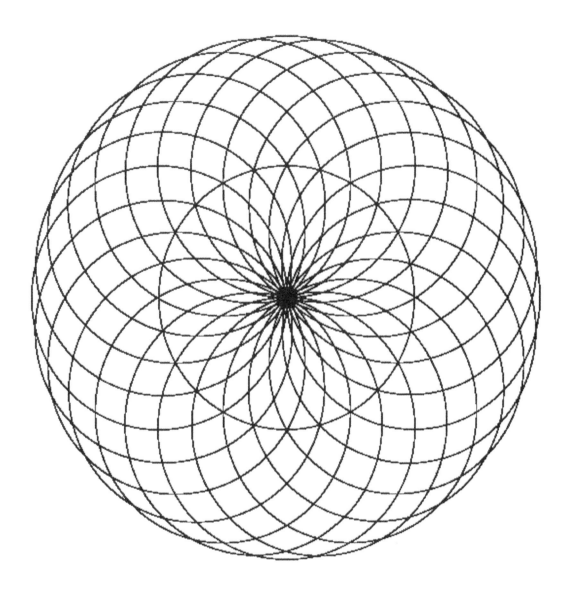

I am free

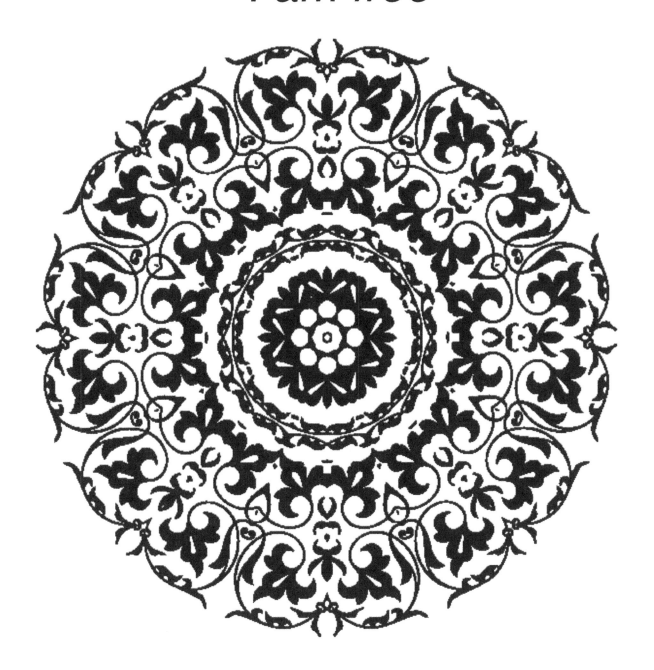

I am stronger now

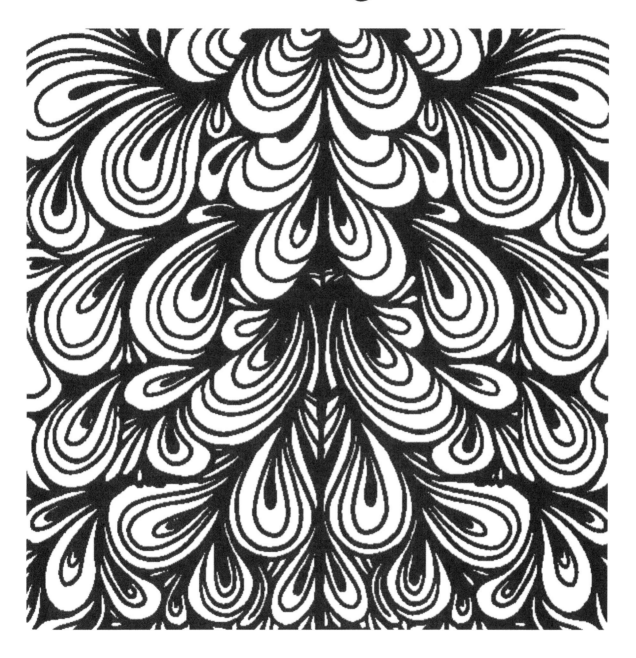

I am a treasure

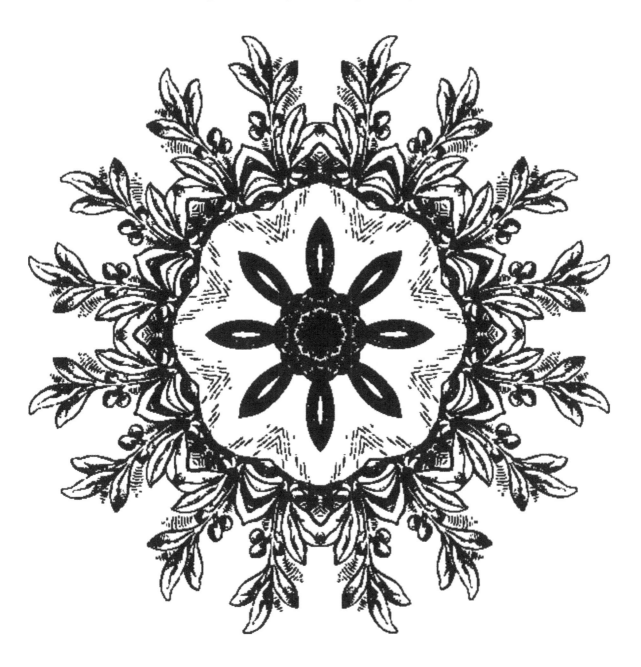

I am capable

I can have love

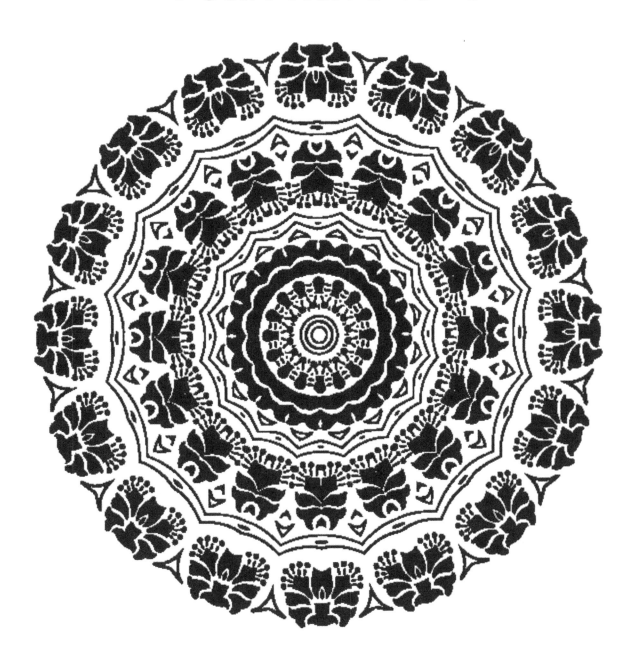

I am attractive

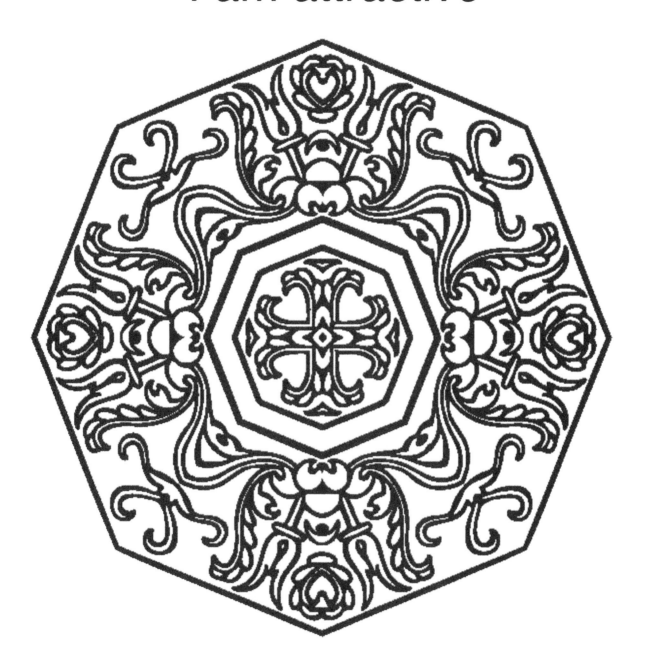

I am fine

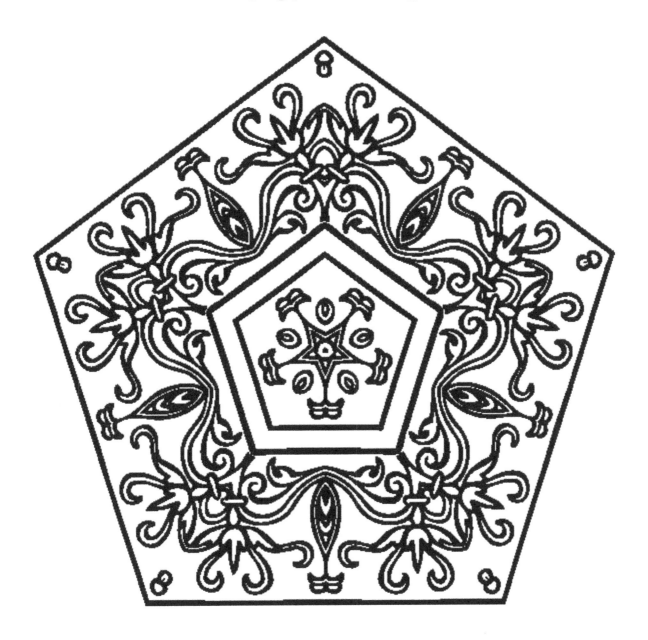

It is over

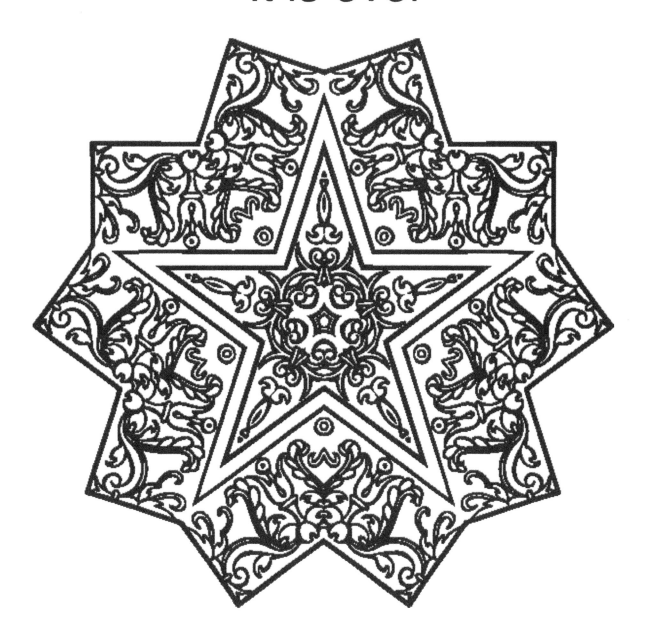

I am a loving person

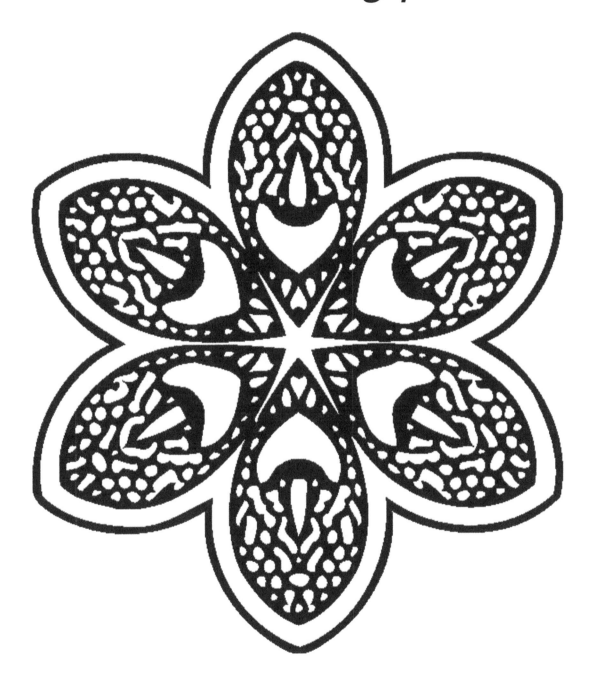

I am justified

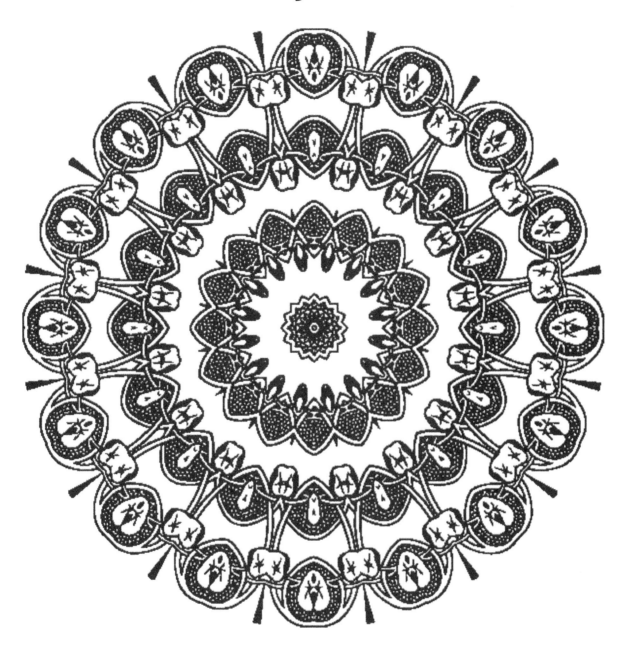

I can let go

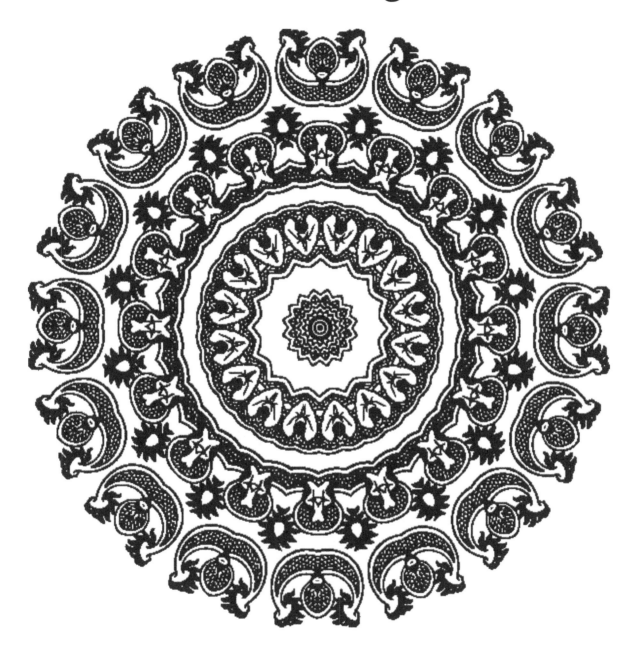

I deserve to be happy

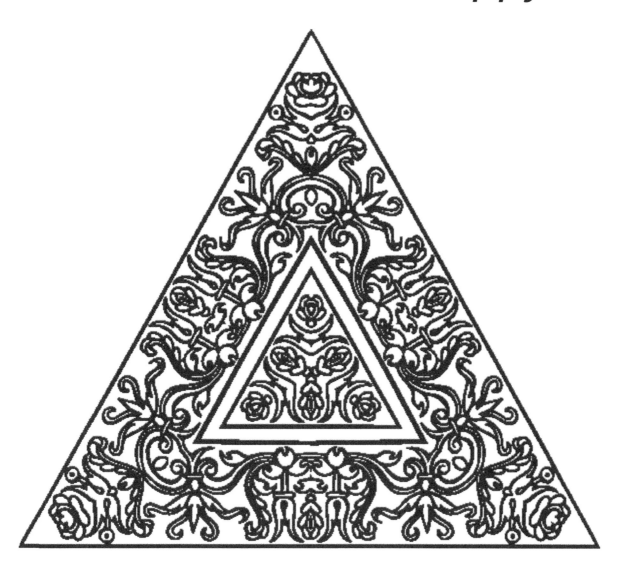

I can become stronger

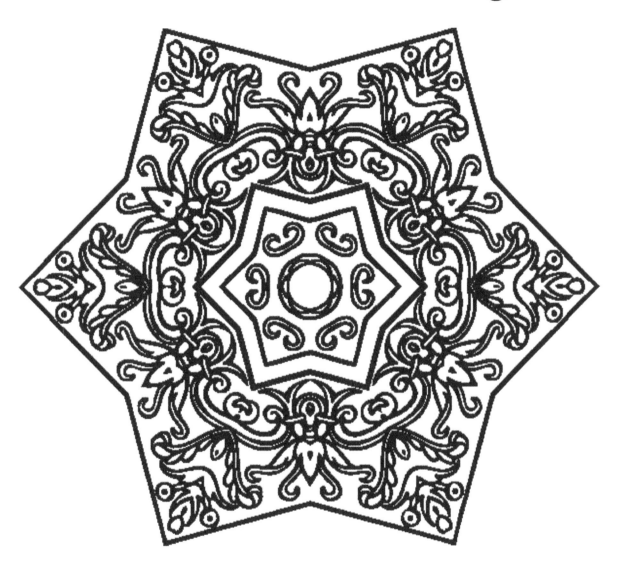

I can trust myself

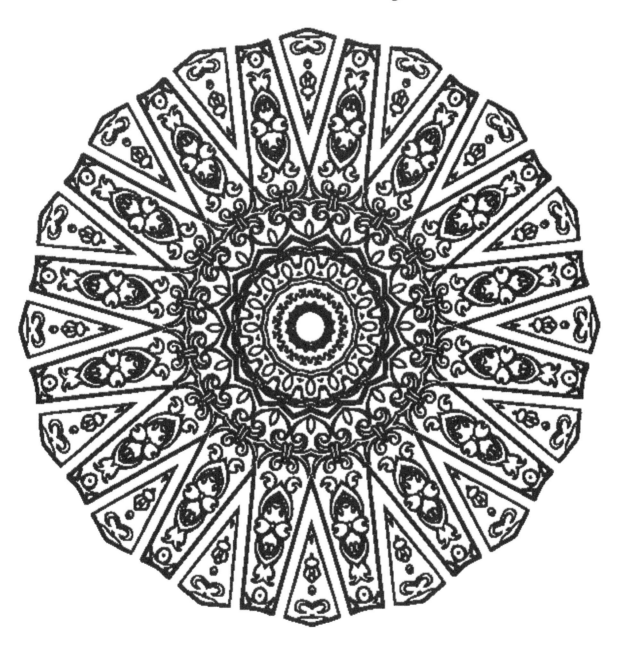

I can succeed

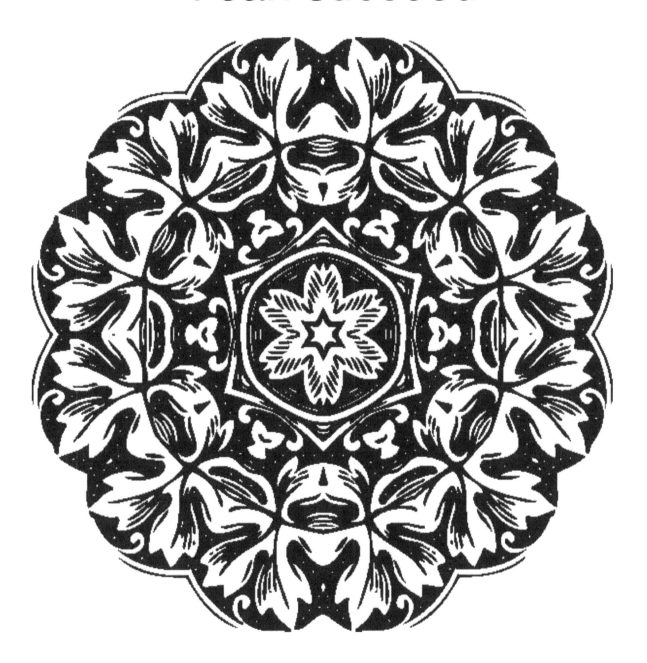

I can choose to let it out

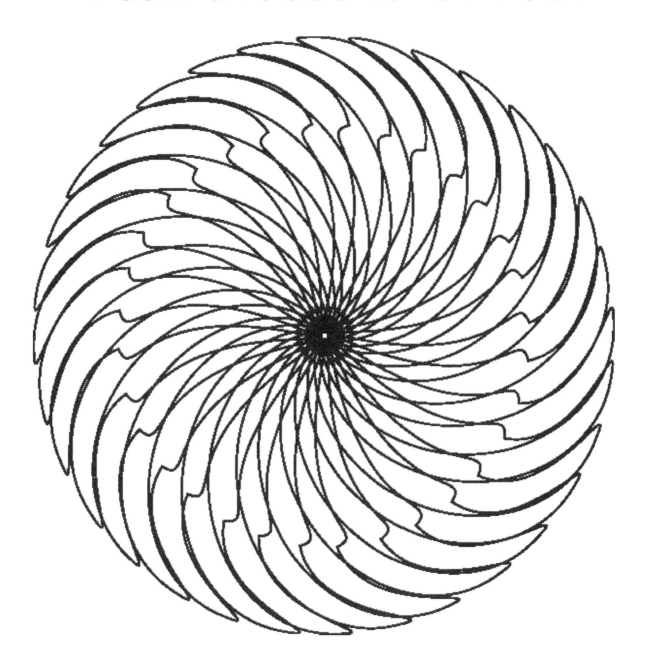

I can take care of myself

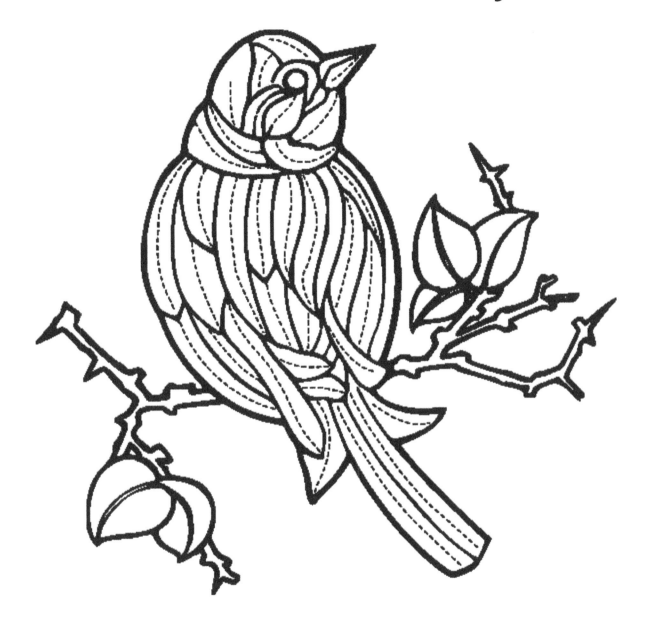

I am important

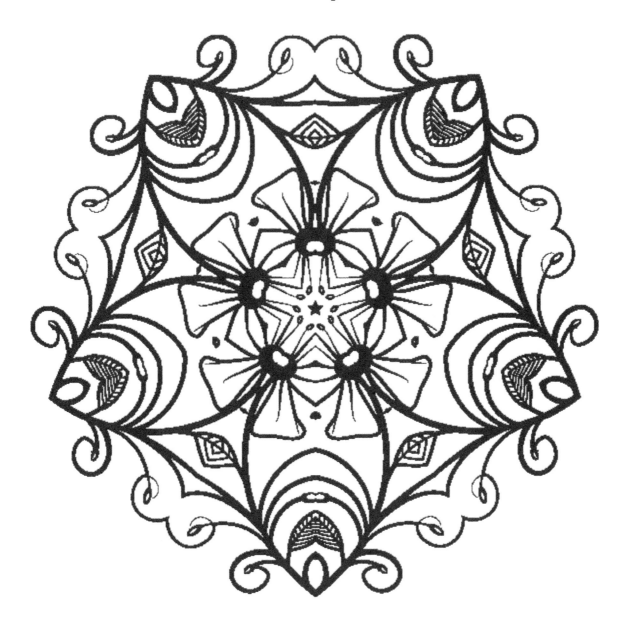

I can make my needs known

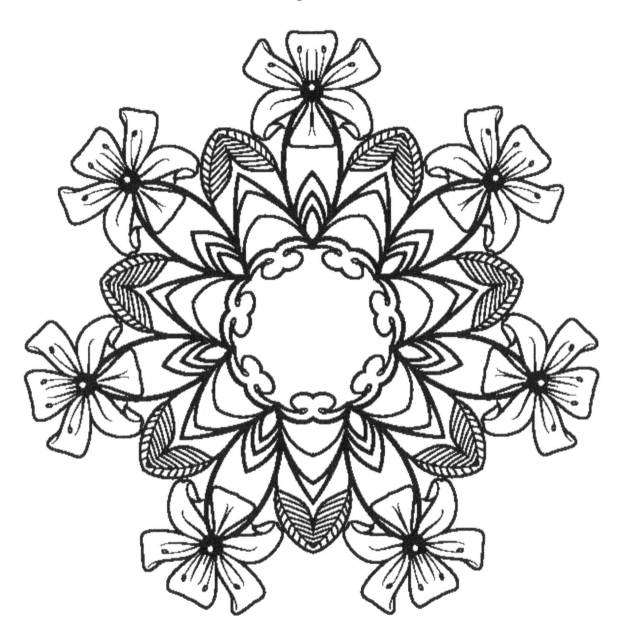

I can choose whom to trust

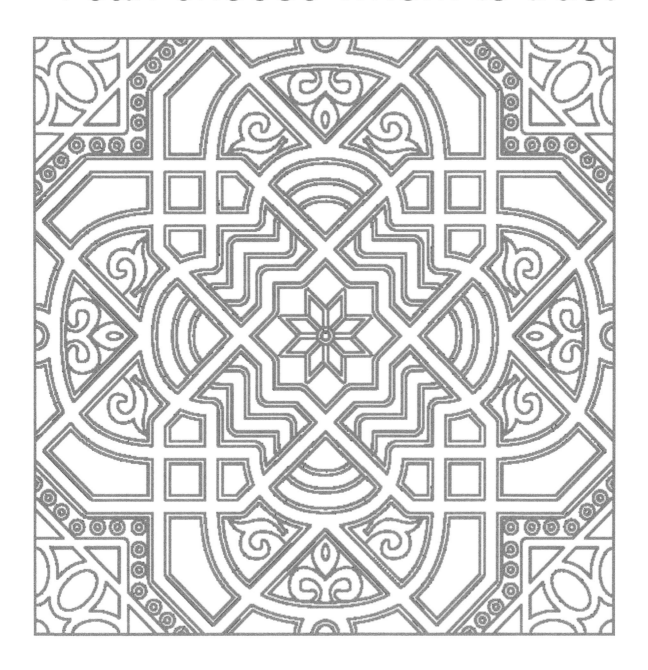

I can be real

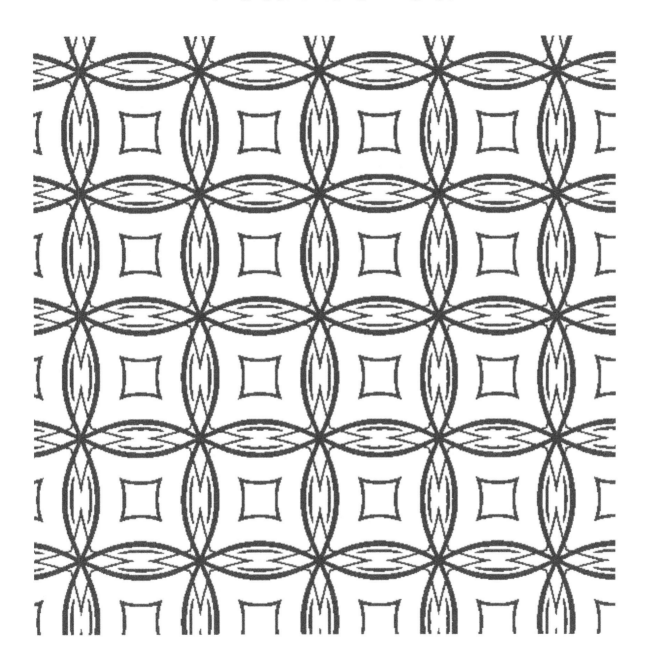

I am okay

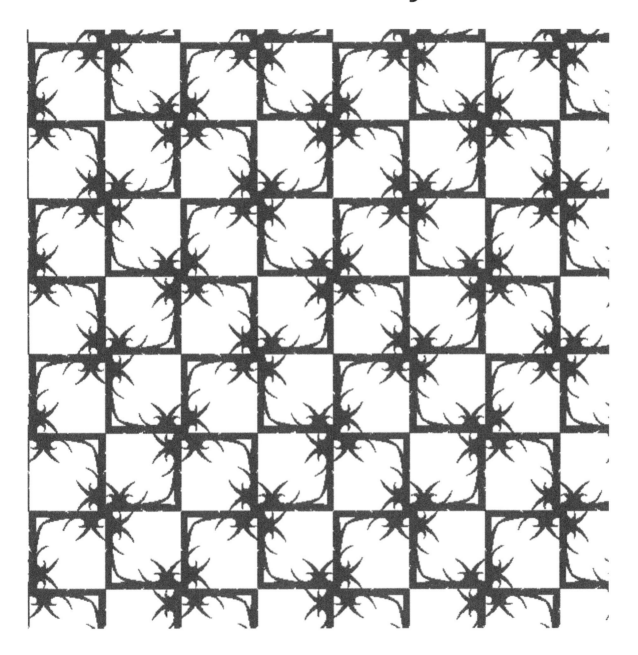

I now have choices

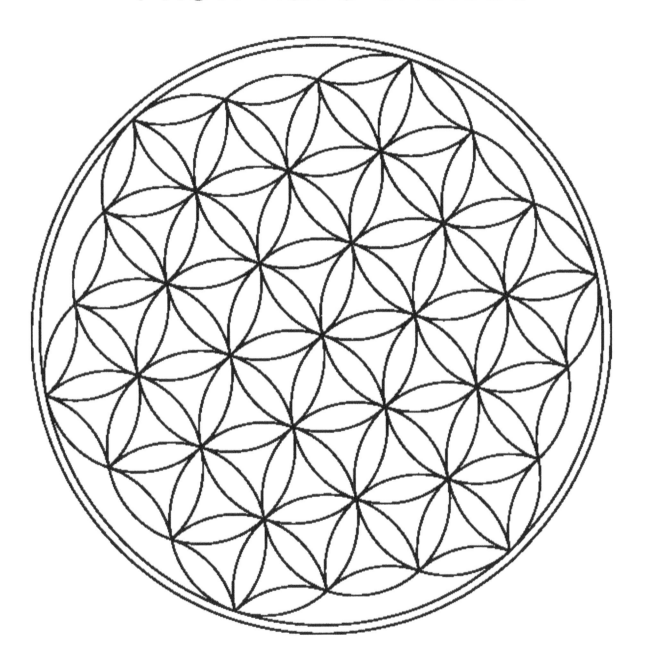

I can take care of myself now

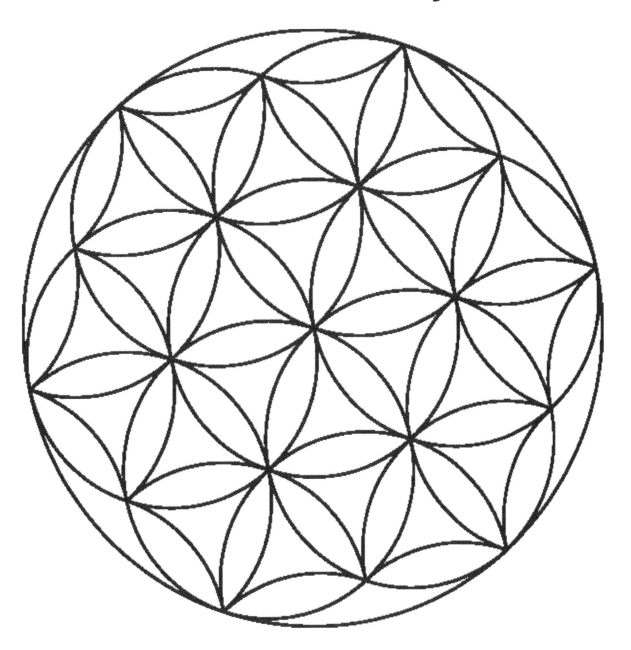

I did the best I could

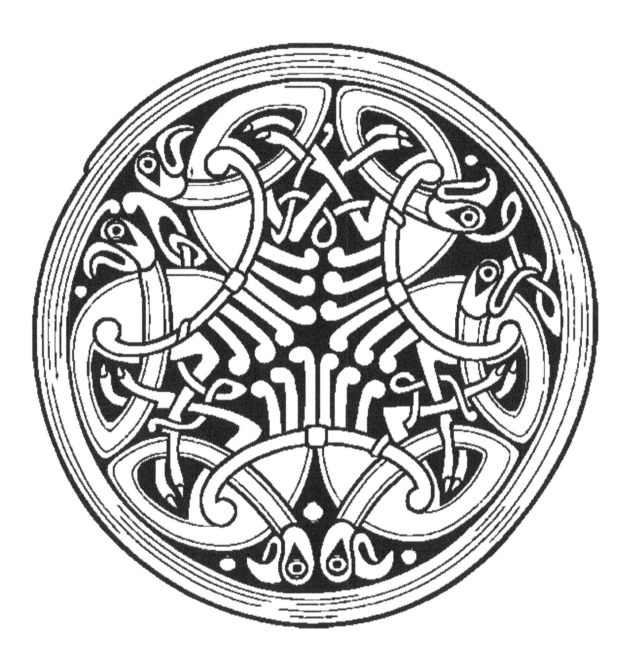

I can learn from it

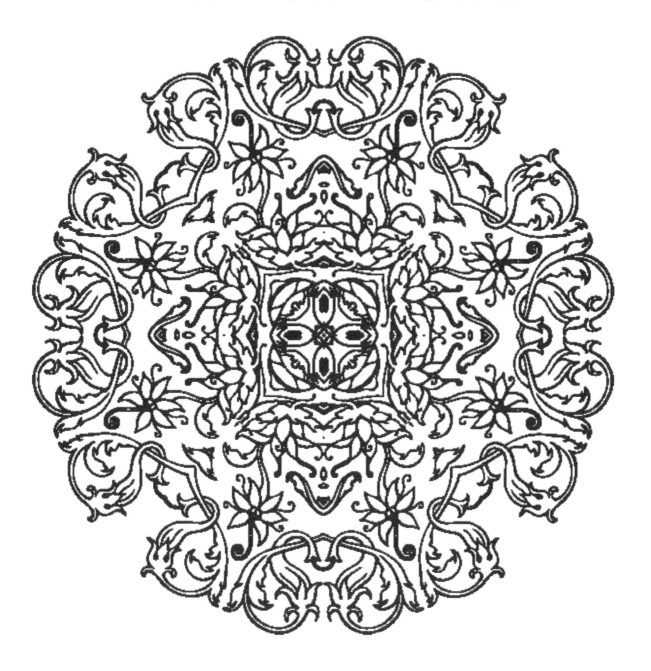

I am lovable

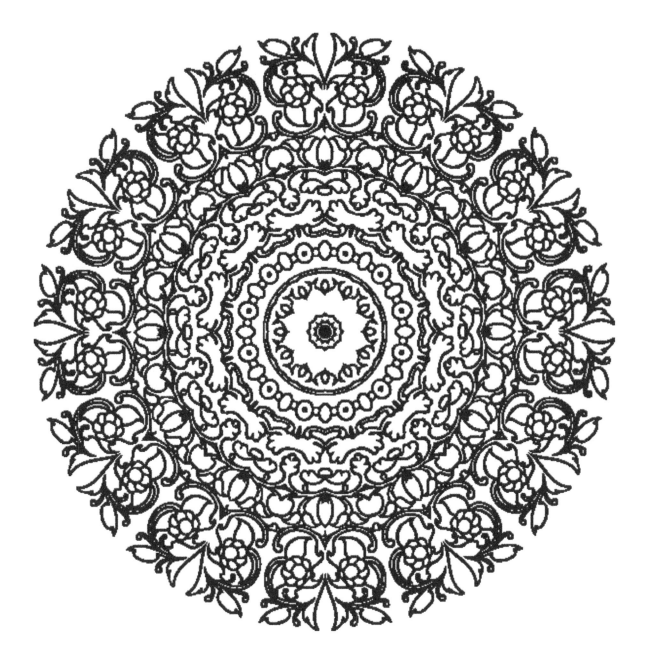

I am beautiful

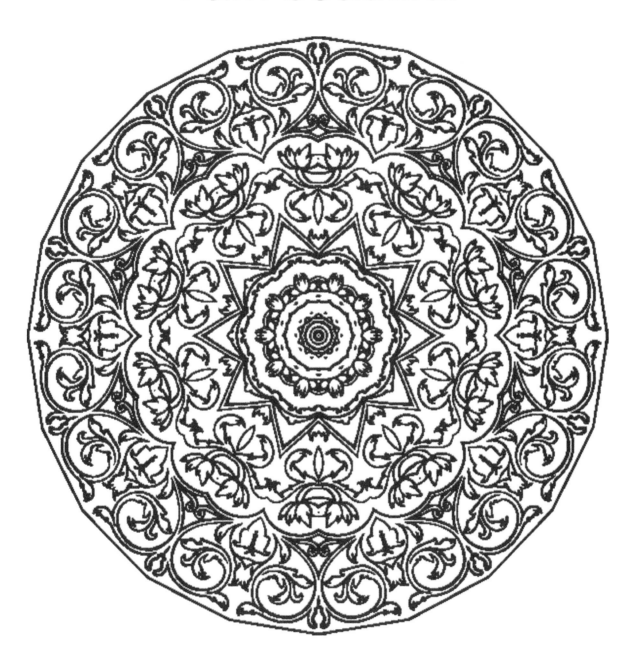

I am significant

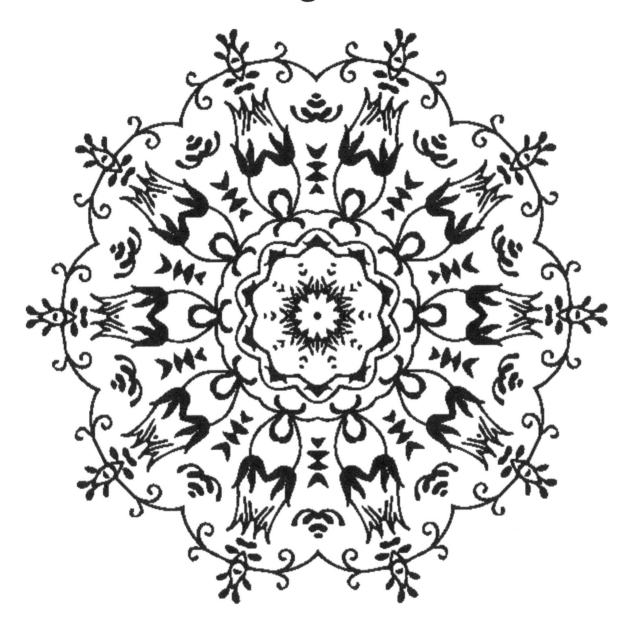

I am worthy of love

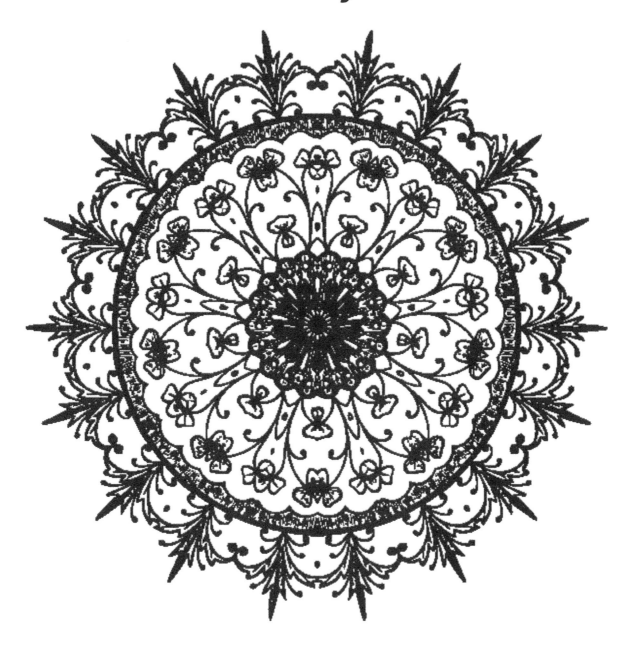

I am precious

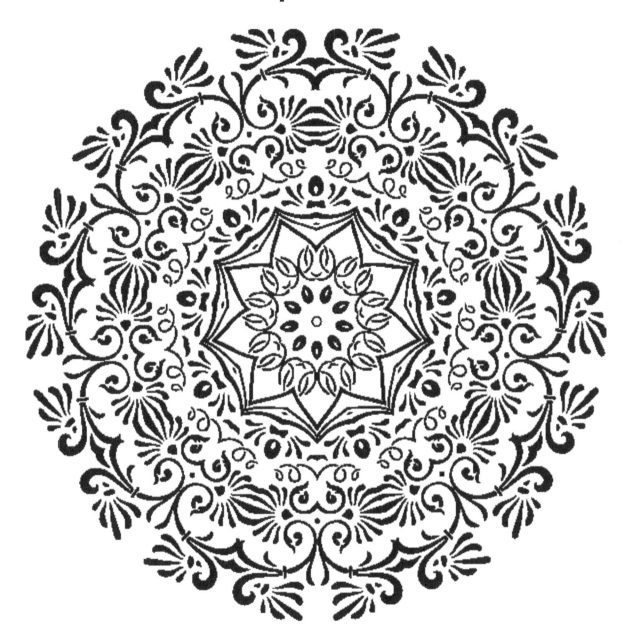

I deserve good things

I can be whole

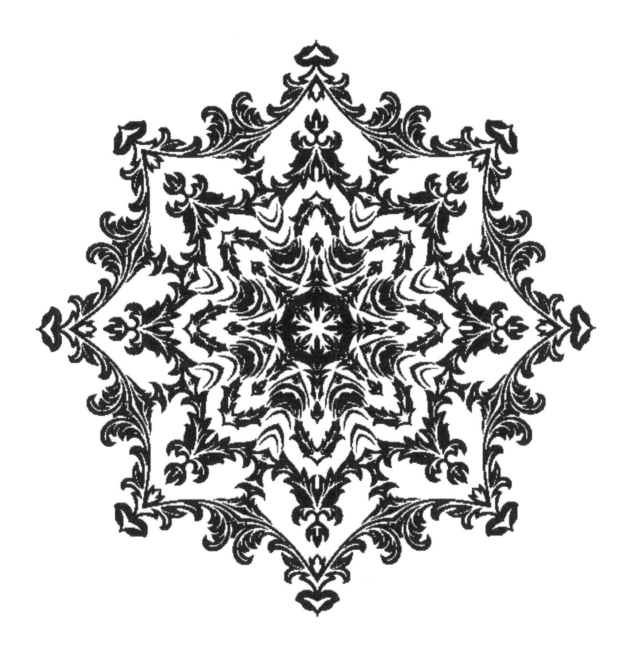

I can express myself

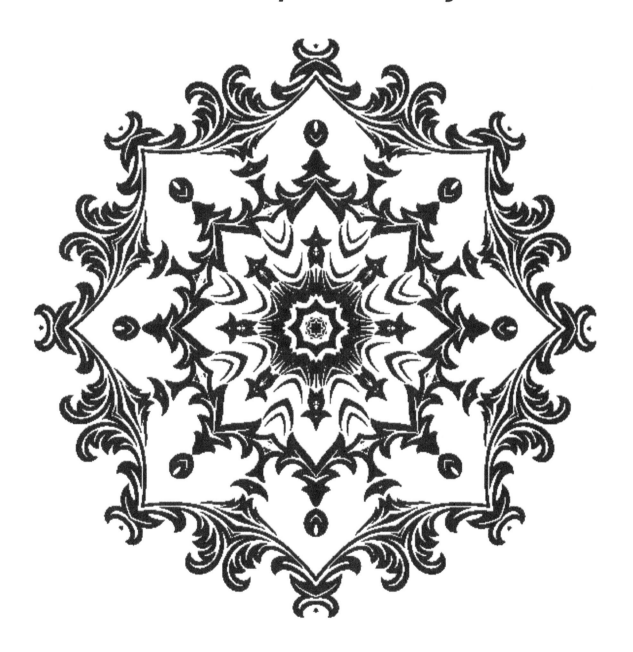

I can live with uncertainty

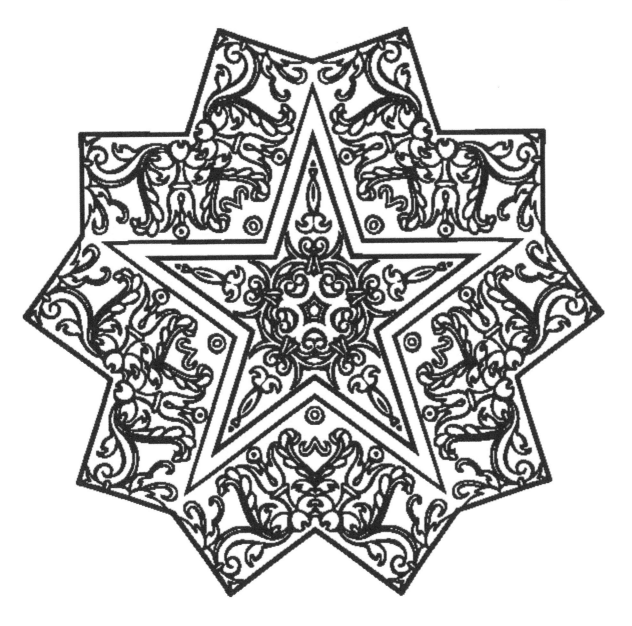

I can grow

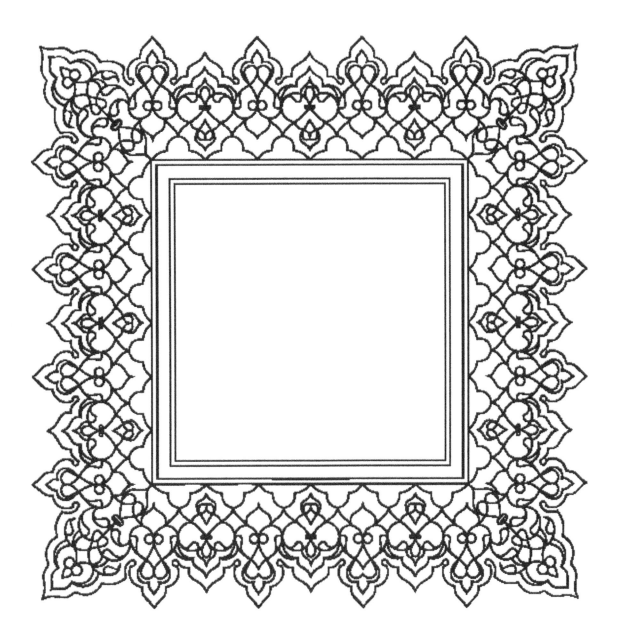

I am worthy

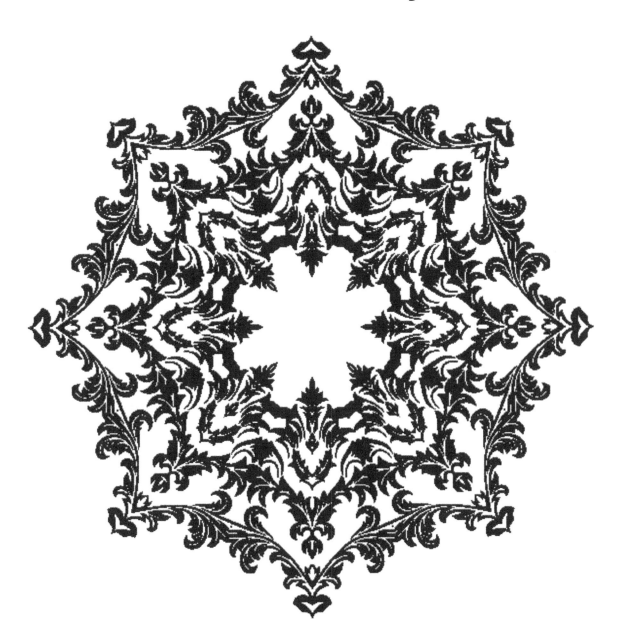

It is finished

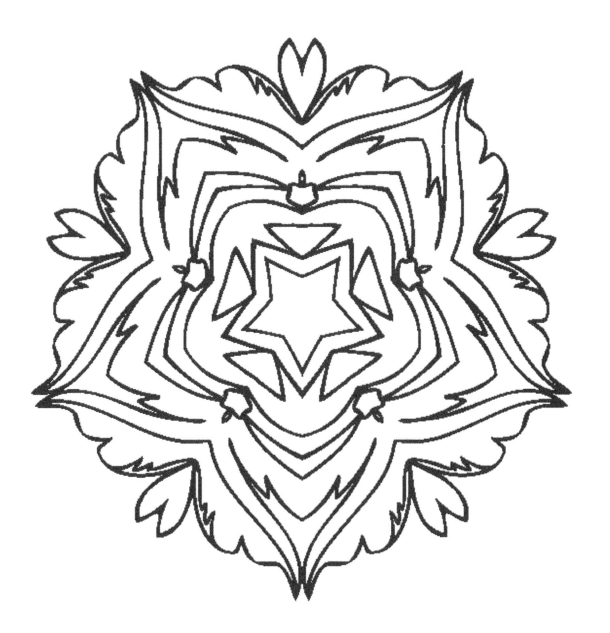

I am radiant

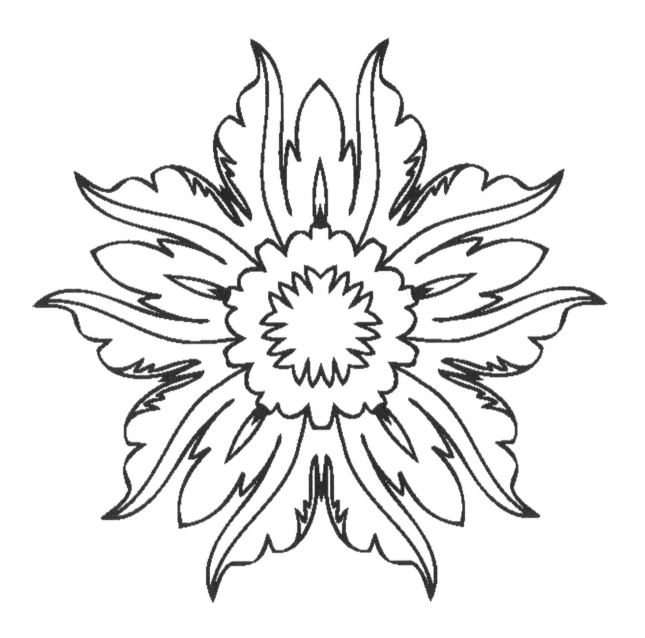

I survived

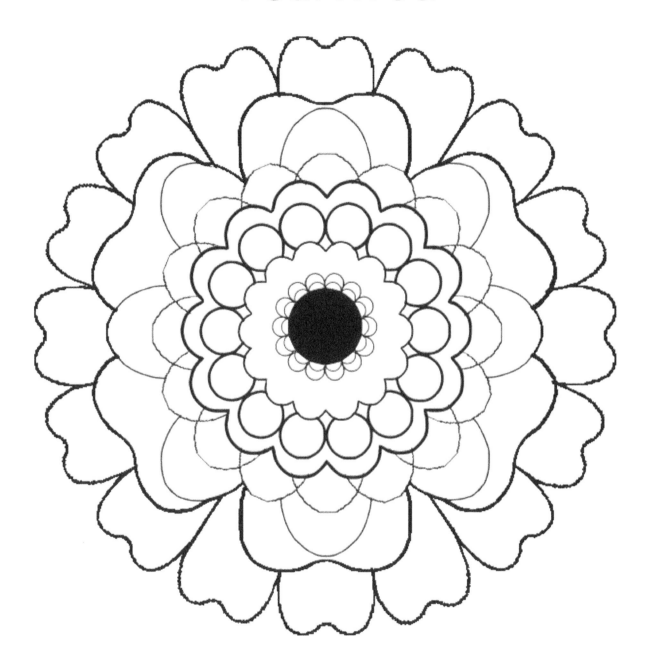

I matter

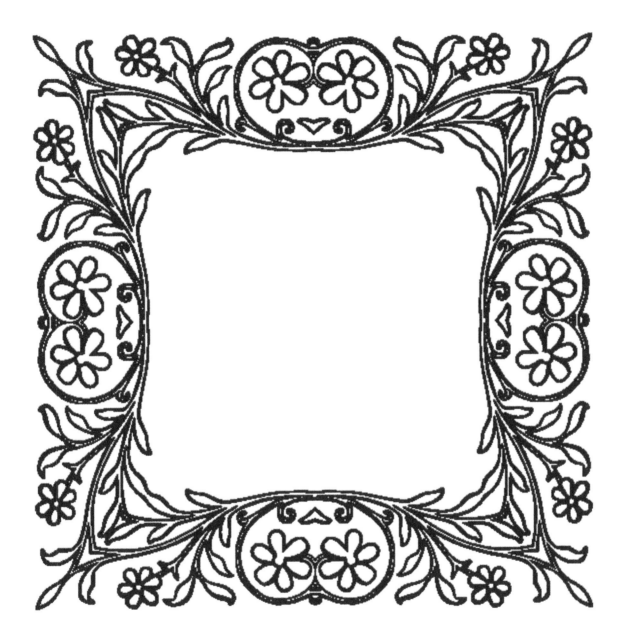

I can trust my judgment

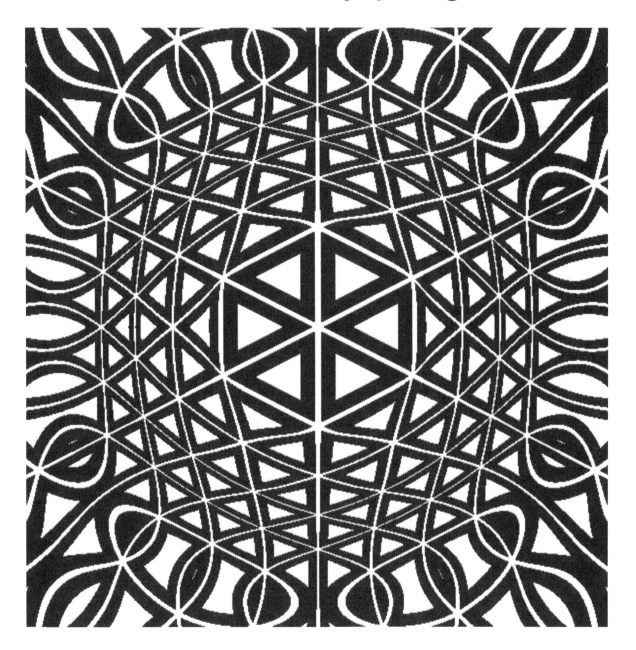

I am safe now

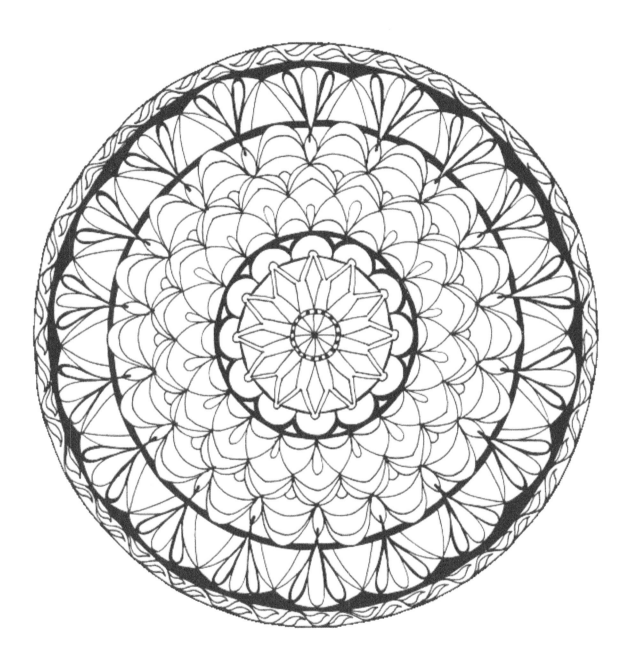

I deserve love

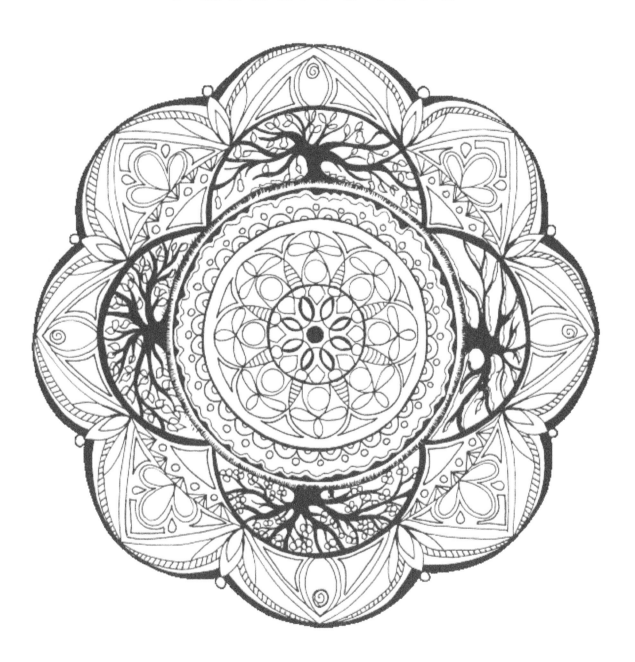

I can be present

I can learn to trust myself

I deserve to live

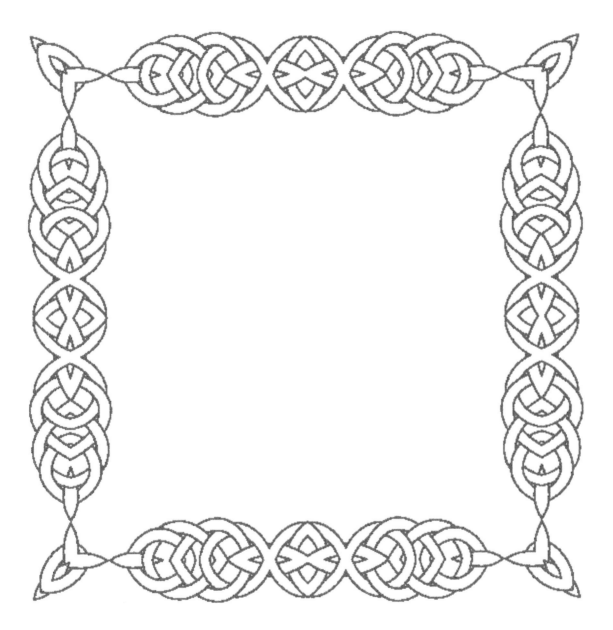

I am not alone

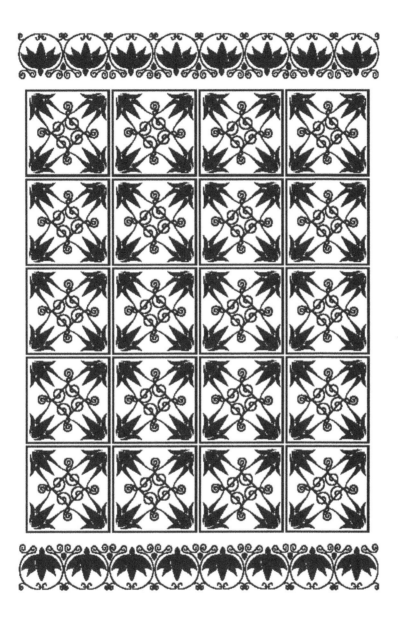

I am able to succeed

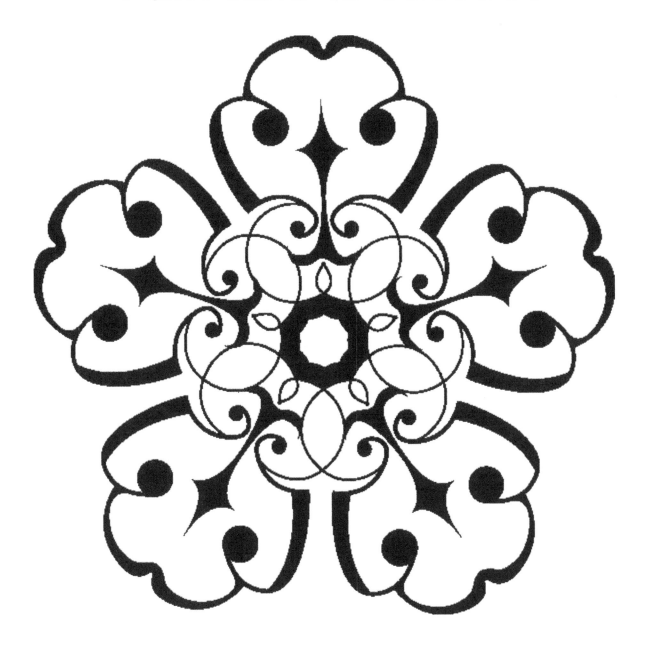

I am worthy of love

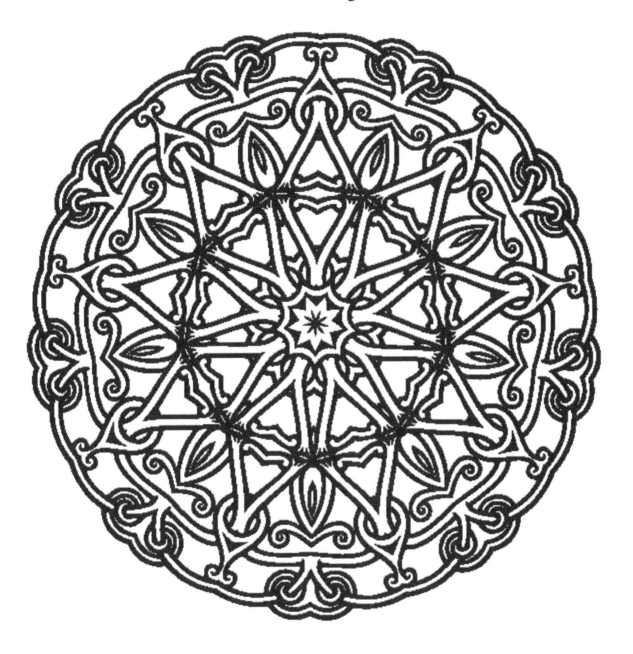

I can be trusted

I am honorable

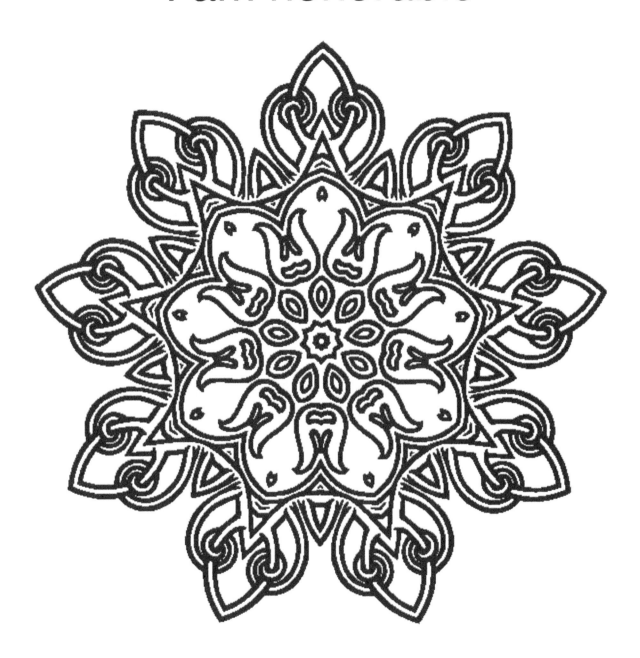

I have dignity

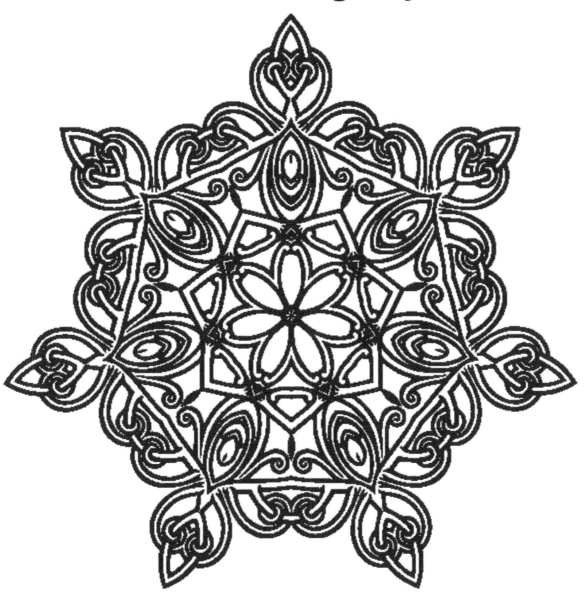

I am valuable

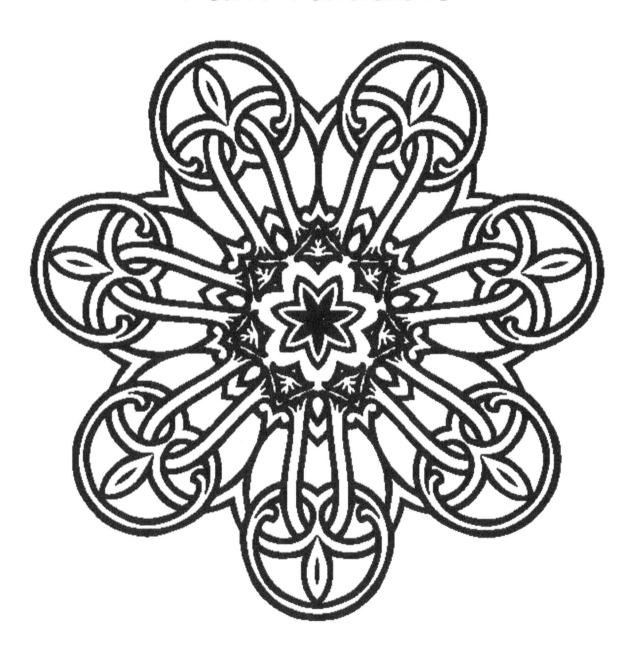

I am stronger than before

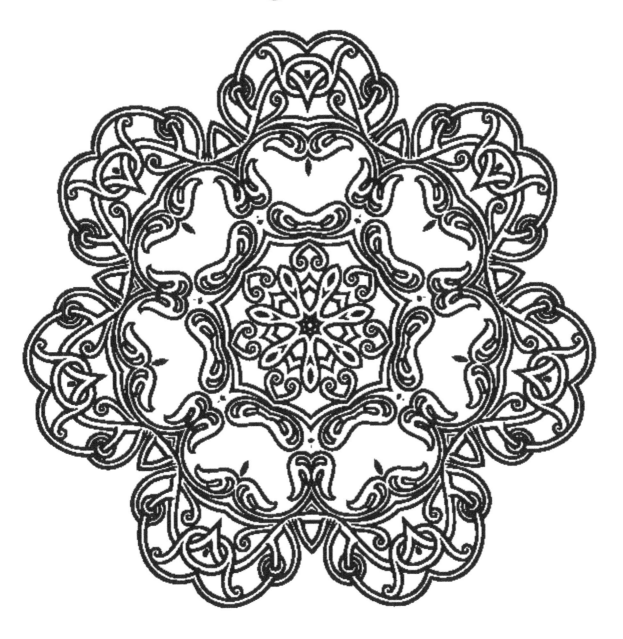

I am fine as I am

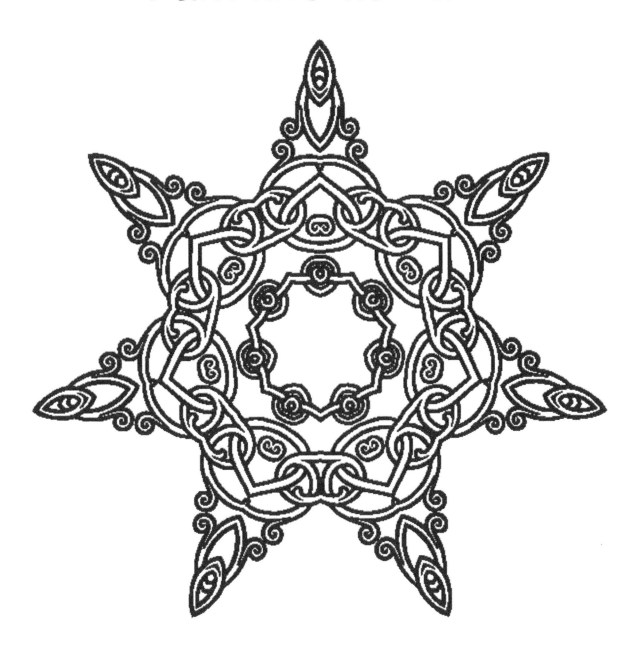

I am only human

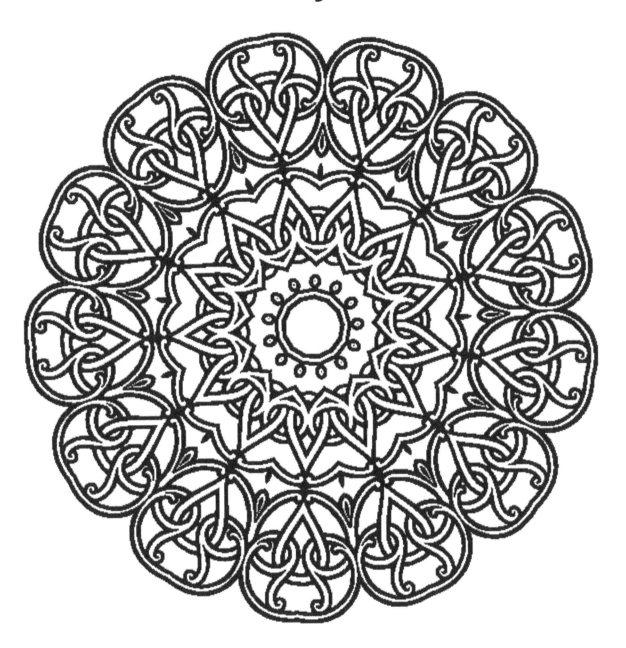

I am smart

I am whole

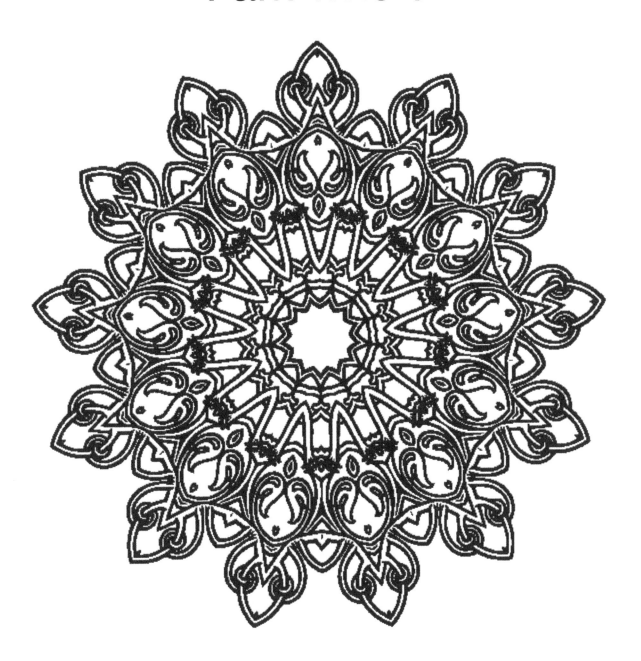

I can handle it

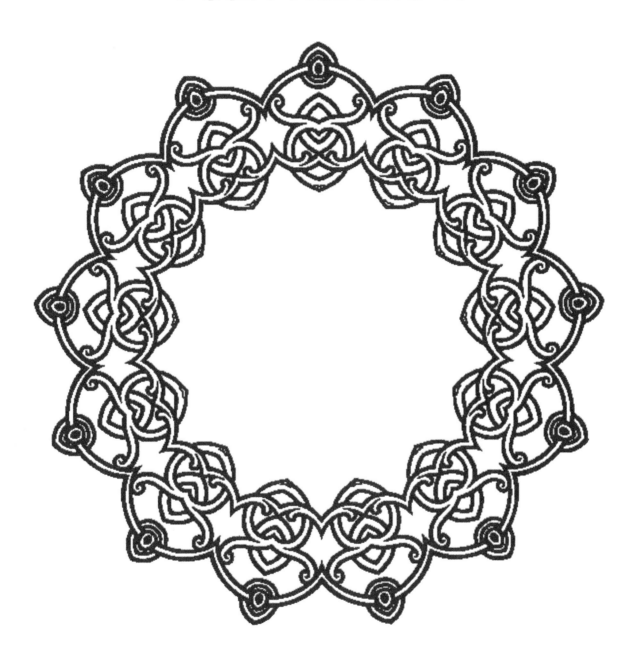

I am enough

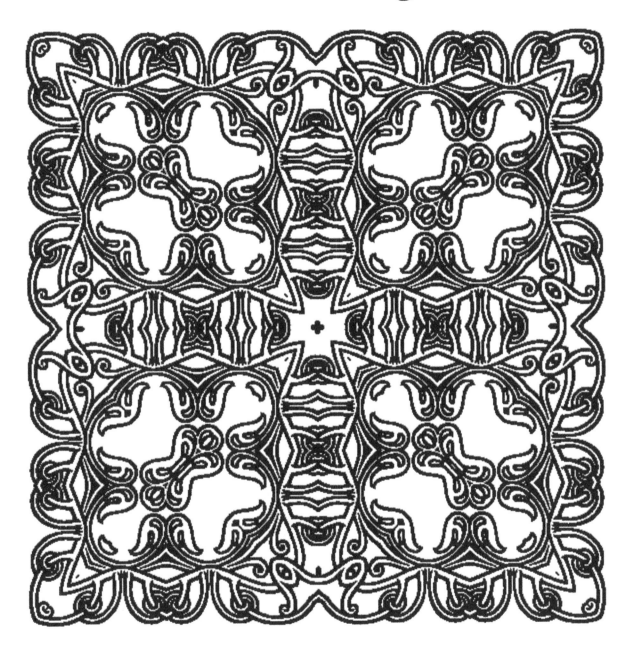

I can be myself

I can make mistakes

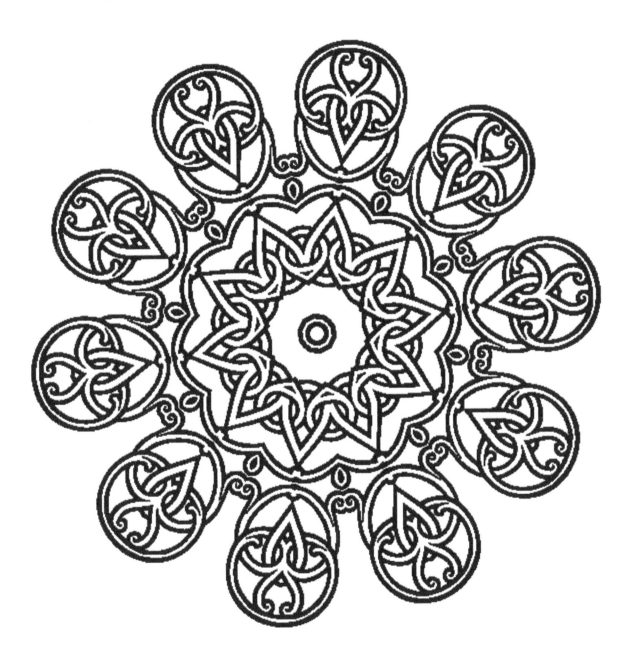

I am intelligent

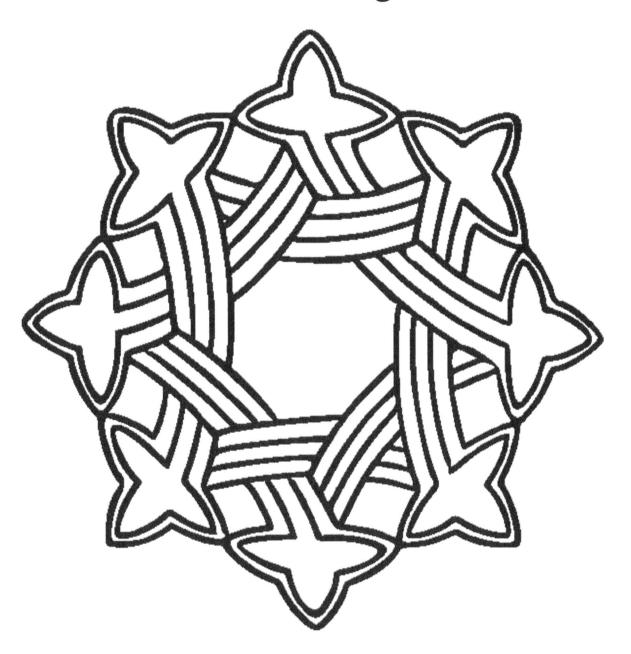

I am strong now

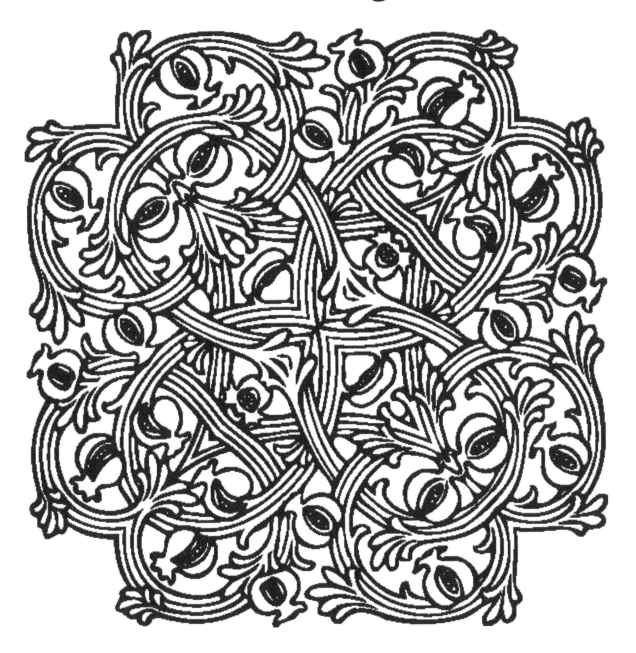

I can be healthy

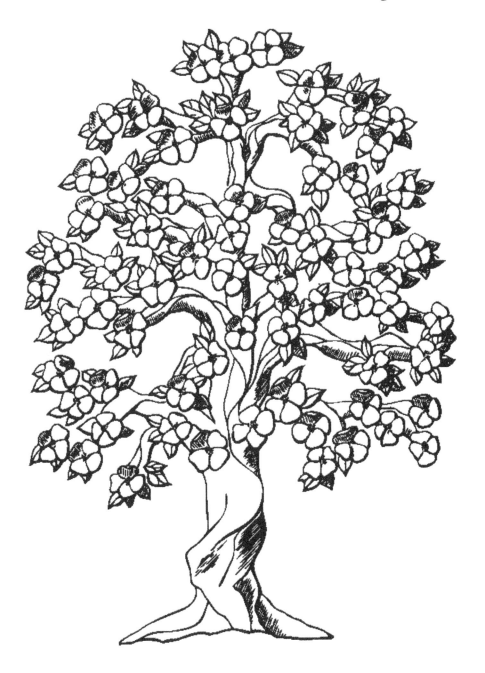

I am a work in progress

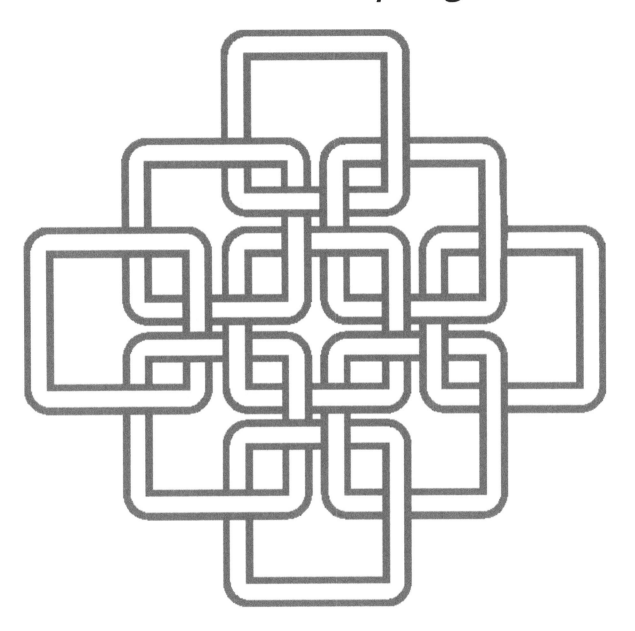

I do the best I can

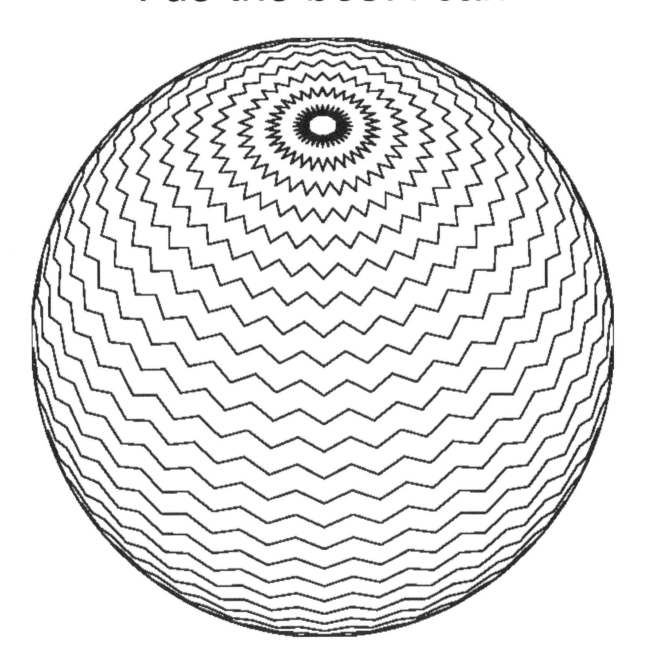

I have been made new

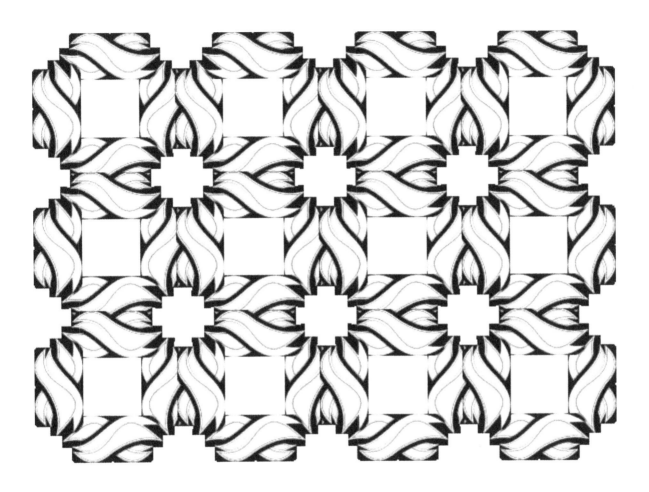

I am okay just the way I am

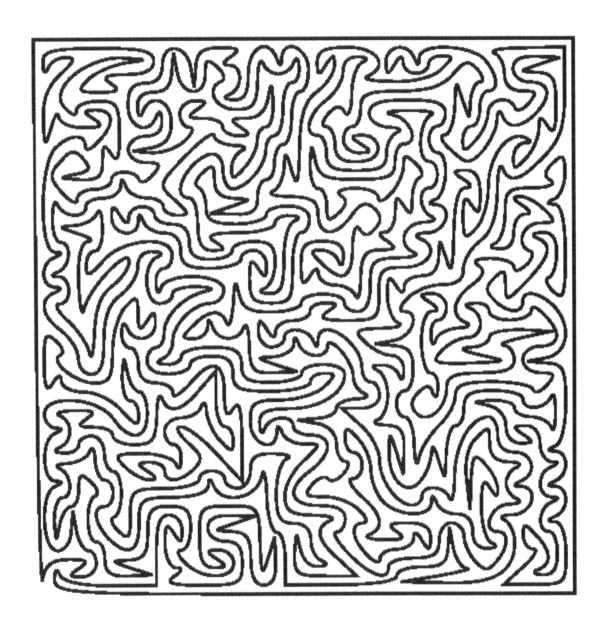

I am strong

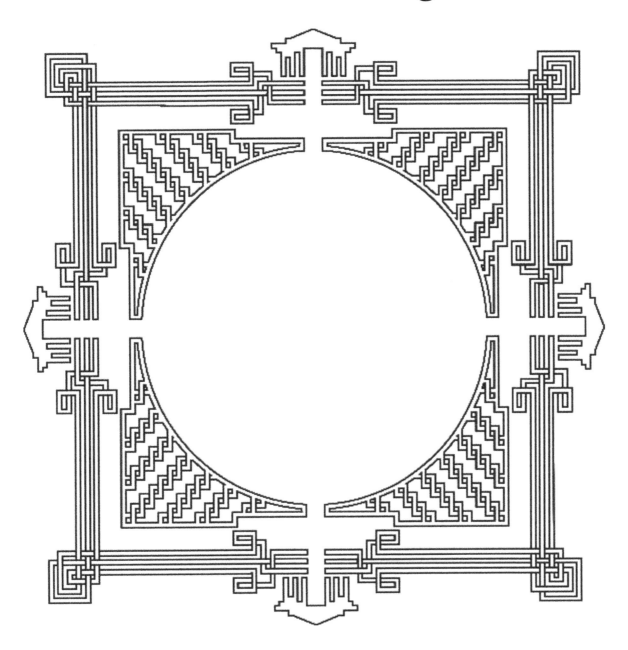

I can do it

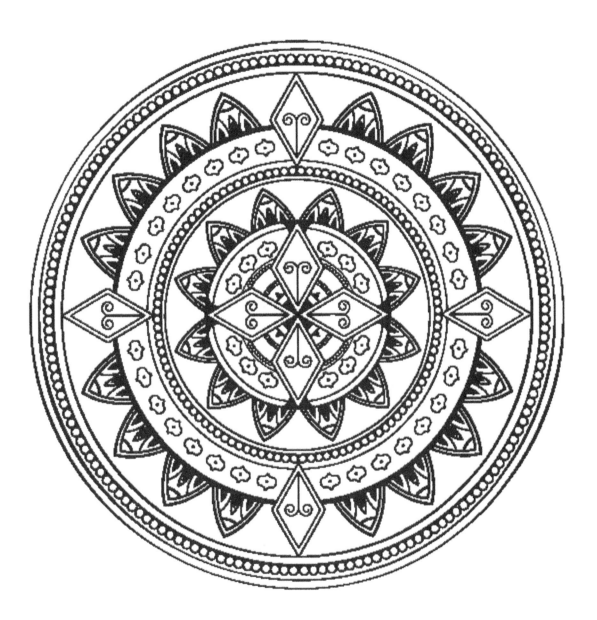

I am forgiven

I have what it takes

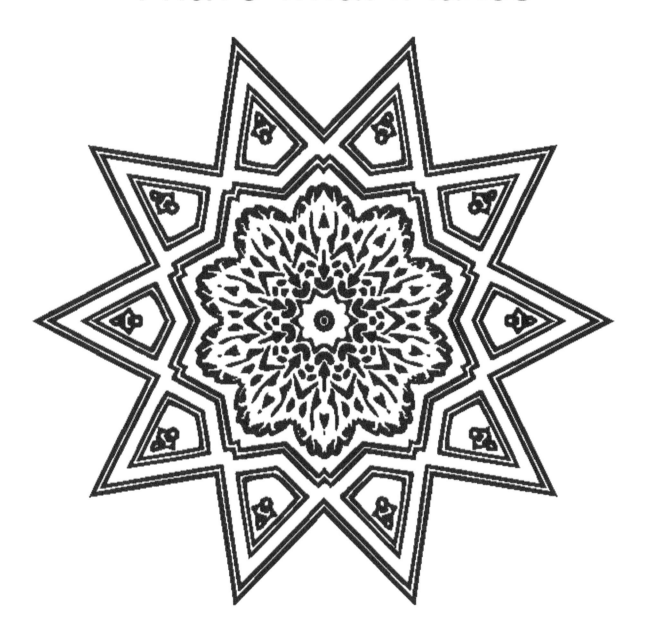

I am okay as I am

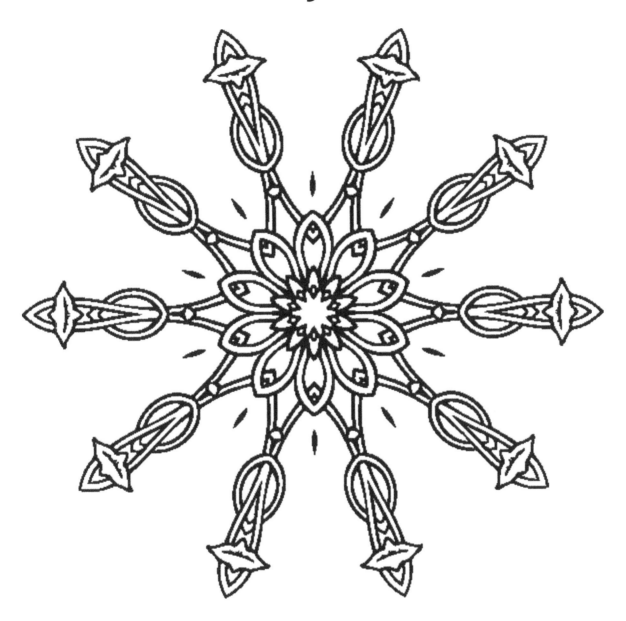

I am a soulful person

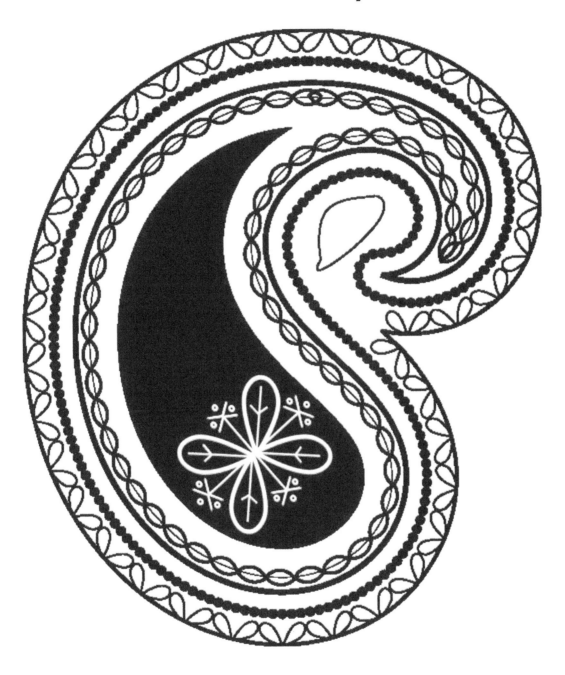

I can accomplish my goals

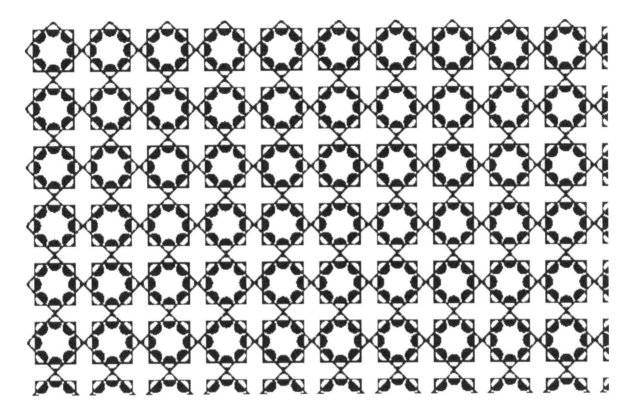

I am valuable the way I am

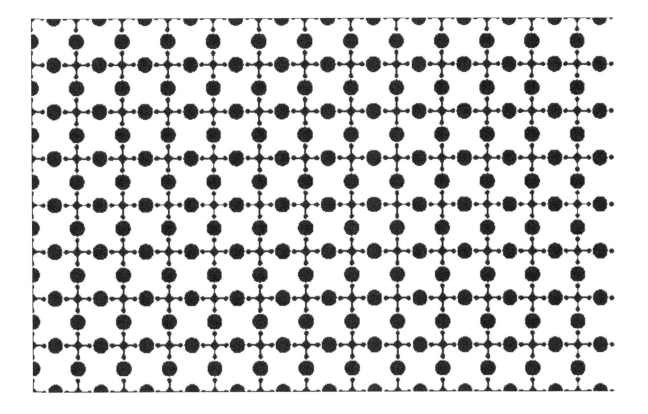

I am not defined by my past

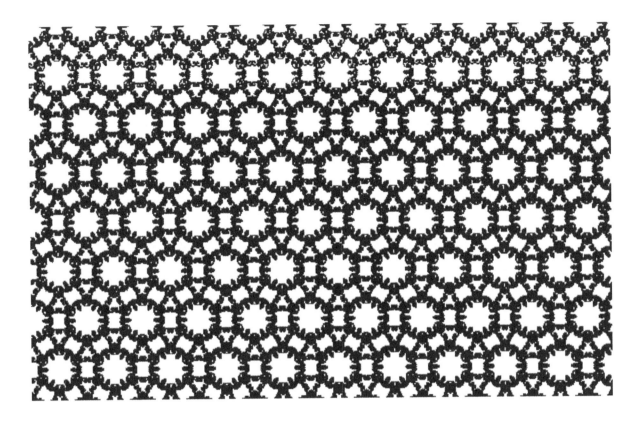

I have mastery

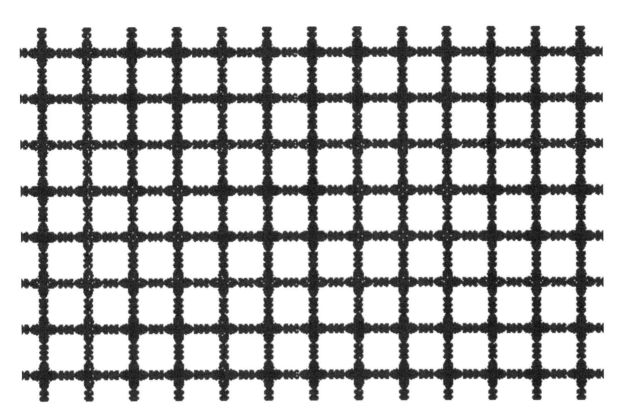

I did enough

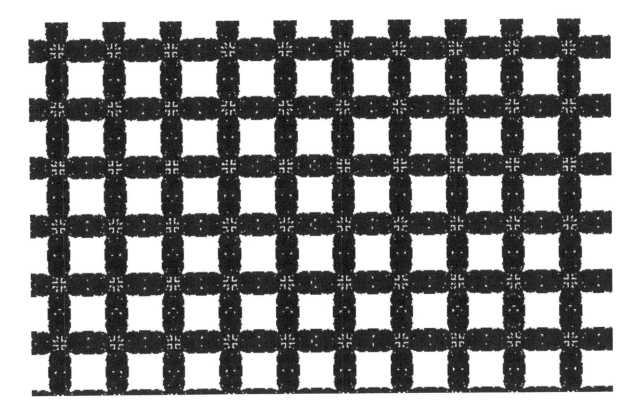

I can be free

I can make good decisions

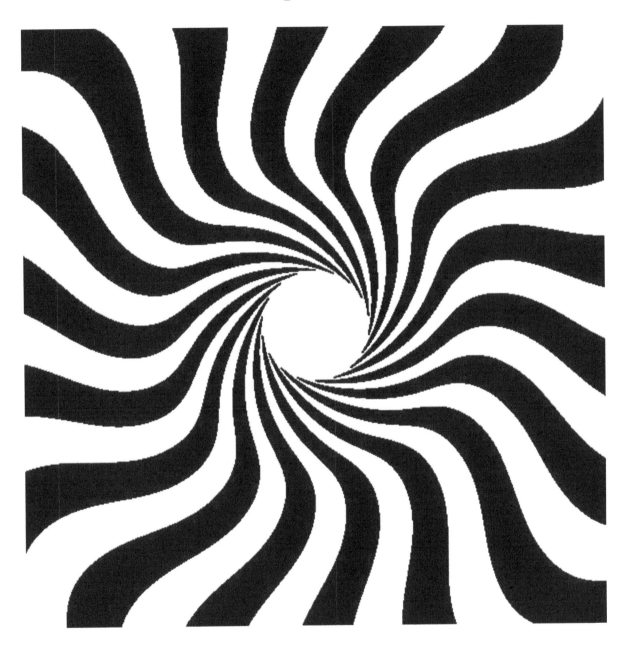

I am alright

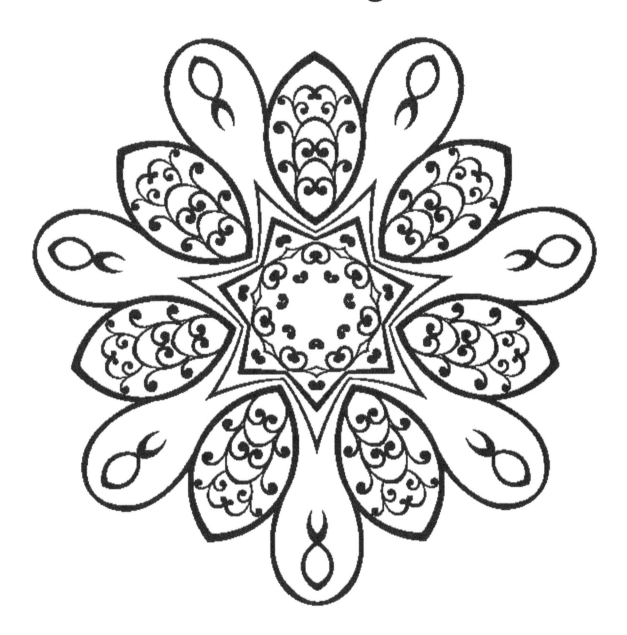

I am lovely

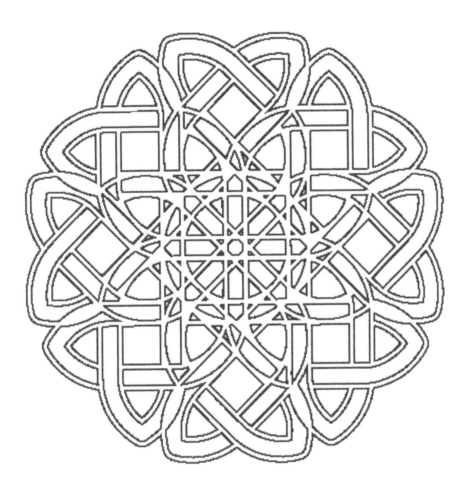

I am remarkable

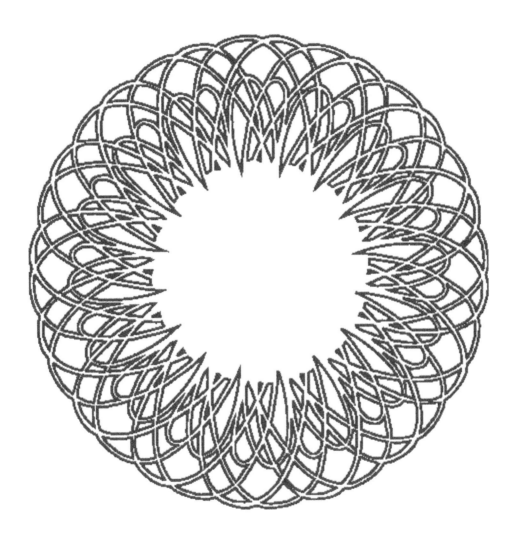

I was just a kid

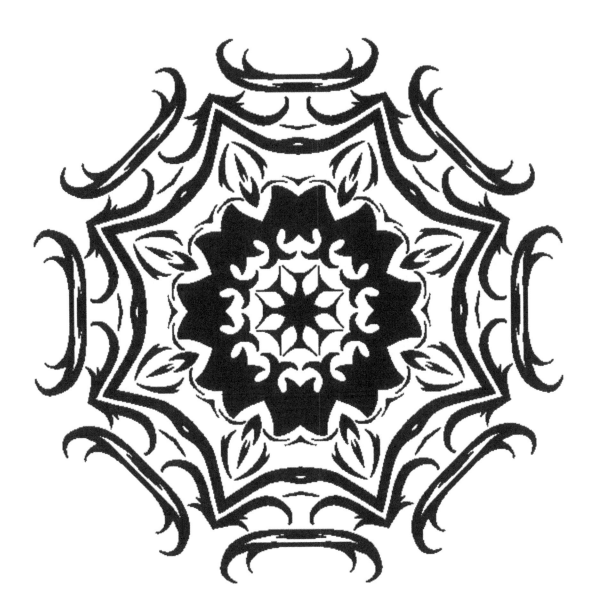

I am stronger now

I can move on

I am able

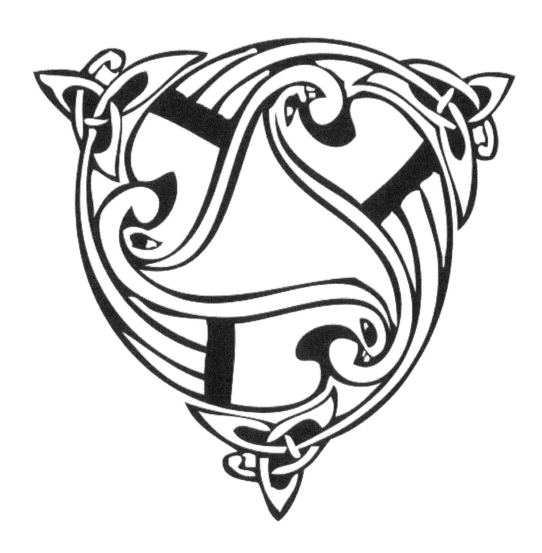

I can conquer my fears

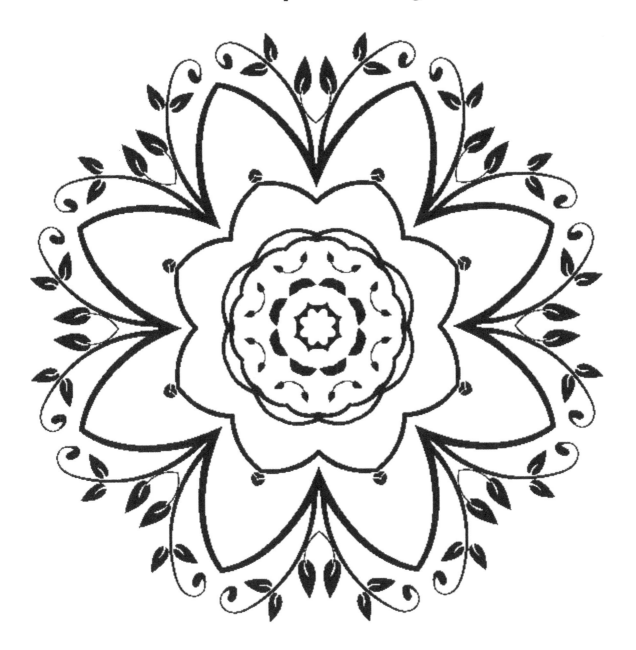

I am a masterpiece

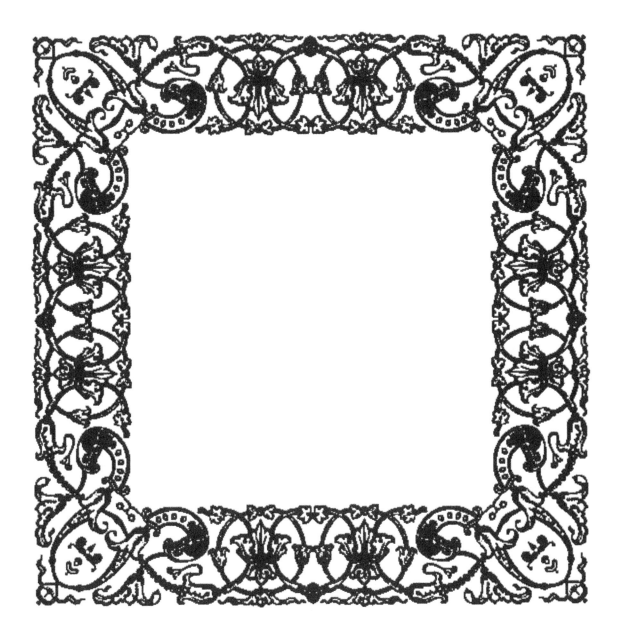

I am a person of integrity

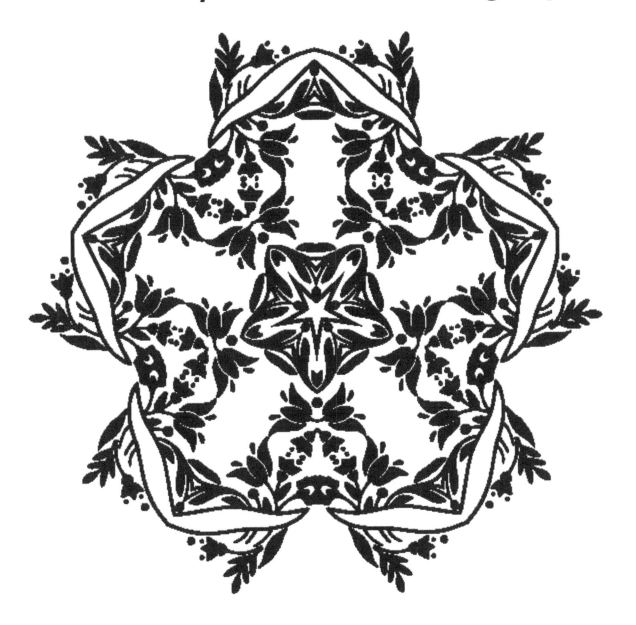

I am priceless

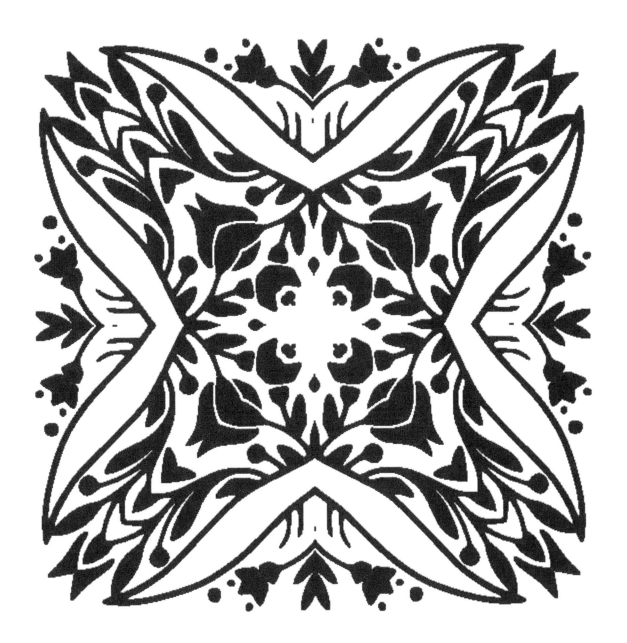

I am respectable

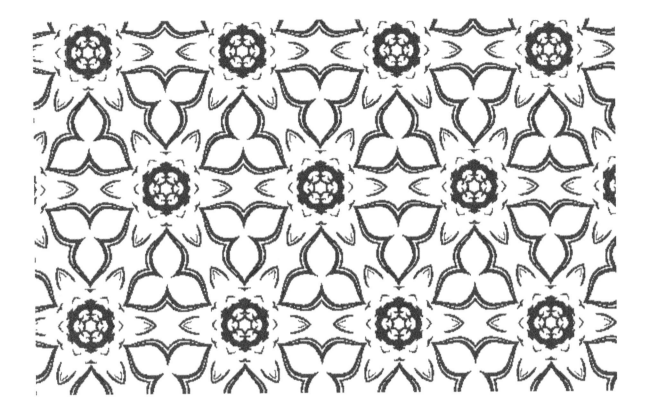

I am a work of art

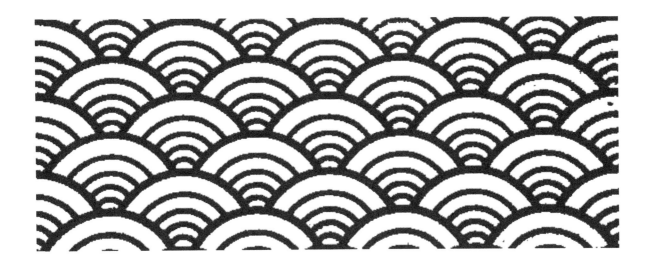

I deserve to thrive

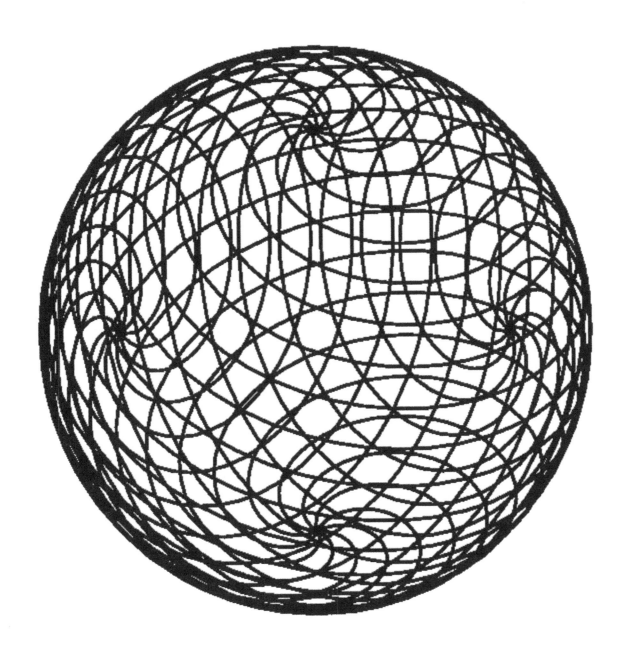

I am okay in my imperfection

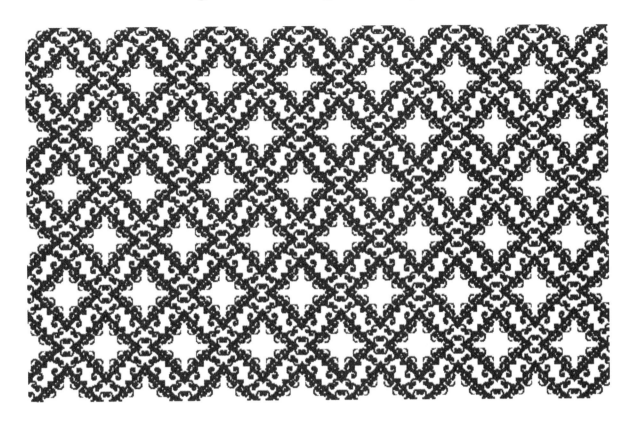

EDITOR BIO

Mark Odland graduated from Augustana College in Sioux Falls, SD, with a B.A. in art and religion. Here he studied drawing, painting, and printmaking under nationally-renowned printmaker Carl Grupp. He went on to earn his M.Div. degree from Luther Seminary in Saint Paul, MN, and his M.A. in Marriage and Family Therapy from the Minnesota School of Professional Psychology in Eagan, MN. An award-winning artist, Mark feels privileged to have his work displayed in various collections around the world. In his work as an EMDR therapist, consultant, and educator, he continues to explore the dynamic intersection between creativity and healing.

CONSULTATION

Mark Odland is able to provide approved consultation for those desiring to:

1) Become EMDRIA Certified
2) Complete EMDR Basic Training
3) Become an Approved Consultant
4) Discuss Difficult Cases

Mark's education, experience, and ongoing training allow him to provide guidance on a variety of issues during consultation sessions. However, he specializes on the following within EMDR therapy: general practice, spirituality, creativity, childhood abuse and neglect, addiction, and military veterans.

CONTINUING EDUCATION

Mark's Odland's continuing education courses are often available as webinars, books, e-books, and audio books. Available to therapists worldwide, his growing list of learning opportunities includes the following subjects:

1) EMDR and Visual Art
2) EMDR and Spiritual Trauma
3) Spiritual Interweaves
4) Spiritual Resource-Building
5) How to Start a Trauma-Focused Private Practice
6) EMDR and Natural Medicine

SPREAD THE WORD

If you enjoyed this book, Mark would be grateful if you left an online review at amazon.com

PURCHASING BOOKS FOR CLIENTS

If you're an EMDR therapist and would like to purchase more copies for clients, you may qualify to receive a discount for bulk purchases. To find out more, send an email to: mark@bilateralinnovations.

PURPOSE

Mark founded Bilateral Innovations with the following purpose:

Bilateral Innovations provides EMDRIA-Approved Consultation and Continuing Education, for the purpose of transforming the world, one client at a time.

To learn more, please visit his website at: bilateralinnovations.com

Made in the USA
Monee, IL
01 September 2021